Productivity and Performance Management in Health Care Institutions

A publication sponsored by the Healthcare Information and Management Systems Society, the American Society for Healthcare Human Resources Administration, and the Committee on Personal Membership of the American Hospital Association

AHA®

American Hospital Publishing, Inc.,
a wholly owned subsidiary of the
American Hospital Association

Library of Congress Cataloging-in-Publication Data

Productivity and performance management in health care institutions

    Edited by Mark D. McDougall, Richard P. Covert,
and V. Brandon Melton.
      Bibliography: p. 175
      1. Hospitals—Administration.
2. Hospitals—Labor productivity. I. McDougall, Mark D.
II. Covert, Richard P. III. Melton, V. Brandon.
IV. Healthcare Information and Management Systems Society.
V. American Society for Healthcare Human Resources
Administration. VI. American Hospital Association.
Committee on Personal Membership. [DNLM: 1.
Efficiency. 2. Personnel Administration, Hospital.
3. Personnel Management—methods. WX 159 P9635]
RA971.P77 1988   362.1'1'0683   88-7869
ISBN 1-55648-027-X

Catalog no. 088166

© 1989 by American Hospital Publishing, Inc.,
a wholly owned subsidiary of the
American Hospital Association.

Printed in the U.S.A.

AHA is a service mark of the American Hospital
Association used under license by American Hospital
Publishing, Inc.

Text set in English Times
3M–12/88–0225
2.5M–3/90–0261

NWST
IAEH 5202

Richard Hill, Project Editor
Linda Conheady, Manuscript Editor
Marcia Bottoms, Managing Editor
Peggy DuMais, Production Coordinator
Marcia Vecchione, Designer
Brian Schenk, Books Division Director

Contents

About the Authors

Raymond A. Buttaro is director, Applied Management Systems, Inc., Burlington, Massachusetts.

Alan J. Goldberg is president, Applied Management Systems, Inc., Burlington, Massachusetts.

James A. Landry is a consultant and health care practice leader, The Wyatt Company, Boston, Massachusetts.

Mark D. McDougall is associate director, Healthcare Information and Management Systems Society, American Hospital Association, Chicago, Illinois.

John A. Page is director of management services, Children's Hospital, Columbus, Ohio.

Vinod K. Sahney is vice-president, corporate planning and marketing, Henry Ford Health Care Corporation, Detroit, Michigan. He is also professor of industrial engineering and operations research, Wayne State University, Detroit, Michigan.

Francis L. Ulschak is director of education, H. Lee Moffitt Cancer Center and Research Institute, Tampa, Florida.

Gail L. Warden is president and chief executive officer, Henry Ford Health Care Corporation, Detroit, Michigan.

John P. Werner is a consultant in Delran, New Jersey.

Glenda M. Westbrook is corporate vice-president, human resources, Hillcrest HealthCare System, Tulsa, Oklahoma.

Foreword

When the Board of the American Hospital Association focused on the need to help hospitals address productivity in today's pressure-filled environment, it was logical to turn to the AHA's 16 personal membership groups for assistance. Responding to the AHA Board's request to develop practical ways to initiate and maintain hospitalwide productivity programs, the central Committee on Personal Membership identified the Healthcare Information and Management Systems Society (HIMSS) and the American Society for Healthcare Human Resources Administration (ASHHRA) to take the lead in developing a resource book for health care institutions. The other personal membership groups, working through the Committee on Personal Membership, provided valuable input into the final product. Leaders in HIMSS and ASHHRA have provided us with a book that is unique in the field.

We are especially proud of this book because it represents the best thinking of practitioners who "practice what they preach" every day. Like its twin, quality of patient care, hospital productivity begins with an overall executive management commitment nourished by a corporate culture that ensures efficiency and effectiveness throughout every hospital department and function.

We trust that readers will discover a gold mine of information and strategies in these pages as they approach a timeworn topic with fresh insights in enhancing patient care.

Edward J. Bertz
Vice-President
Personal Membership Groups
American Hospital Association

Preface

In today's extremely competitive environment, productivity is everyone's business. Hospitals are faced with shrinking bottom lines, growing competition, and, according to many, a significantly increased risk of hospital closure. Hence, it is more important than ever for each hospital employee to perform his or her assigned task in a manner that provides a high-quality product in the shortest reasonable amount of time. Managers and administrators have the additional duty of providing an atmosphere that is conducive to high levels of productivity for all employees.

Responding to the difficulties facing hospitals today, the contributors to this book have set forth multiple strategies for obtaining excellent performance and high levels of productivity. By adopting such strategies, hospital management can take a more aggressive approach to improving the utilization of human resources, the quality of health care services, and the selection and performance of employees.

Utilization of Human Resources

Faced with the infinite number of hurdles that hinder operational productivity improvements, hospitals need to employ those tactics that are most effective in their institutions. For example, the physical environment has a significant impact on productivity, and management must ensure the proper placement of departments, the best location of workstations within departments, and the design of the workstations to effectively and efficiently accomplish the required tasks.

Another tactic is to study the interaction of the departments and personnel in the hospital. The delivery of effective health care services depends on the smooth interactions of many people. However, bottlenecks do occur both between and within departments. Once bottlenecks are identified, management can take steps to eliminate or minimize them.

In addition, staff utilization, including innovations in patient and employee scheduling, needs to be managed better. As each department improves its match between staffing patterns and work load, the utilization of all hospital employees improves. For example, many departments experience distinct fluctuations in work load throughout the shift, day, week, month, or year. By minimizing the peak/valley syndrome typically associated with health care services, the unproductive time of workers can also be minimized.

Likewise, steps can be taken to effectively match staff to work load. It is a fact of life in hospitals that work load usually does not fit smoothly into the typical 7-to-3 or 9-to-5 workday. Therefore, hospitals should seriously consider implementing alternative staffing patterns, such as staggered schedules, four 10-hour days, three 12-hour days for 40 hours' pay, fewer full-time and more part-time employees, and a centralized float pool.

To improve the understanding of resource utilization within a hospital, an effective management reporting system should be instituted. Such a system allows the staff and the supervisors to understand what is happening in their department. The system also allows supervisors to determine the correct number of employees to carry out the functions of the department with a minimum of idle time.

Although productivity improvement efforts have typically focused on operational efficiencies, clinical effectiveness issues are becoming significant factors in many productivity management programs. When physicians reduce unnecessary testing, a hospital's operations become more effective and efficient. One of the roles of top-level management can be to foster the cooperation of the medical staff toward improving clinical effectiveness.

Quality of Service

Contrary to the opinion of many people, high productivity levels do not necessarily mean low quality. If quality is plotted against productivity, the quality will be low at low levels of productivity, broadly peak at a reasonably high level of productivity, and then fall off only when the productivity exceeds the level that is beyond the ability of the average worker to perform. This concept is made on the basis of several factors that have been observed in many industries:

1. People prefer to be busy. Busy workers are happier workers, and such workers tend to make fewer mistakes.

2. People actually do a better job when they are relatively busy. Underemployed workers are more inclined to make errors because their minds are not totally occupied with the work at hand.
3. Workers who are working slower than their natural pace tend to make errors of omission, whereas workers who work faster than their normal pace are inclined to make both errors of omission and errors of commission, which are mistakes in what they do as opposed to what steps they omit.

When taking steps to improve productivity, hospitals can improve quality at the same time. They can measure and manage quality like any other performance characteristic by collecting the right data and using certain analysis techniques described elsewhere in this book. Institutions that do this are likely to find that reasonably high levels of productivity and reasonably high levels of quality can and do occur at the same time. We use the terms *reasonably high levels of quality* and *reasonably high levels of productivity* because it is obvious that if either quality or productivity is pursued to the extreme, the other must suffer. Nevertheless, productivity is not independent of quality; rather, the two are interrelated.

Employment Practices

Productivity is also affected by employment practices. A new employee often is not a highly productive employee. He or she needs time to become used to the organization, the workplace, and the other workers. A new employee can take up to several weeks to reach a satisfactory level of productivity, depending on the complexity of the job. An institution that repeatedly selects unqualified employees or employees ill-suited to their jobs is likely to experience high levels of turnover and, hence, lower levels of productivity.

To reduce the costs of turnover, managers must take great care in selecting the proper person for each job. First, they must recruit only those persons who are technically competent for the position to be filled. Second, they must ensure that each new employee fits with the culture of the organization and is able to stand up to the stress of working under the pressures of a health care work environment. Managers have several ways available to them to assess the suitability of job candidates.

Furthermore, any policy that will nurture and develop existing employees should yield a level of productivity greater than when new employees need to be constantly recruited and trained. Managers must structure the work environment to promote both loyalty and high levels of achievement among existing employees.

Employee Performance

In order to attain high levels of productivity, particularly from supervisors and managers, it is necessary to link incentives to performance. For this reason managers will find it highly desirable to implement a performance management system. Such a system enables an organization to select appropriate techniques for appraising performance and ensuring employee development.

One important role of a performance management system is to set realistic objectives for every employee, thus enabling employees to know what supervisors expect. Such a system also tells workers exactly how they will be rewarded and allows them a chance to know how they are performing. High achievers are workers who get regular feedback, which in turn fosters clarity of role, commitment to the goals of the organization, and a strong sense of purpose in fulfilling day-to-day obligations.

For the top-level manager, productivity measures should be included in his or her evaluation and should be successively incorporated in the evaluation system as one moves down the organizational chart, thus reinforcing productivity measurement as an organizationwide priority. For example, for the department-level supervisor, performance management becomes the primary means of communicating what is expected, and it can often be tied to the productivity of those working for the supervisor. If the productivity of the employees is related to the supervisor's performance evaluation, the productivity of the entire unit will most likely be higher.

The rewards and incentives for productivity must be appropriate and meaningful and can be both monetary and nonmonetary. Monetary incentives can be most effective, particularly over a short time frame, and increasing attention is being paid to incentive programs (such as variable pay programs) for all employees. This is in reaction to the swiftly rising costs of employee benefits, which are forcing employers to look for alternatives to the more traditional methods of compensation.

For supervisors and management, many institutions are currently using long-term as well as short-term incentives, all of which are tied to performance evaluations. Although long-term incentives have normally been offered first to top-level management, they are being extended more and more to the lower levels of the organization.

Recognition and reward can also take the form of greater benefits and perquisites and such nonfinancial rewards as earned time off, flextime, and office amenities. Many ways exist for employers to show their appreciation for improvements in productivity. Whatever is valued can be used as a reward, whether the reward is directly linked with increases in productivity or whether the increase in productivity is a secondary effect of having a more enthusiastic employee.

Administrative Commitment: A Critical Requirement

Successful productivity improvement and performance management efforts all have one major common attribute: complete support from top-level administrators. It is the responsibility of top-level management to set organizationwide goals and to provide the work environment in which those goals can be reached.

Each administrator influences the institution in more than just giving explicit orders. Administrators set the tone of the organization's culture by how they conduct themselves. Although the culture may have been established before an administrator came to the institution, it can be assessed and changed to conform with his or her concepts of management, service, and employee relations.

Administrators must actively champion strategies that enable management and staff to perform their duties most effectively and efficiently. Without complete support from top-level management, the expected benefits from a productivity improvement effort may be limited. But the effective use of well-thought-out strategies and programs can improve an organization's bottom line and its competitive advantage over other institutions

Mark D. McDougall
Associate Director
Healthcare Information and Management Systems Society
American Hospital Association

Richard P. Covert
Director
Healthcare Information and Management Systems Society
American Hospital Association

Acknowledgments

This project was spearheaded and edited by Mark D. McDougall and Richard P. Covert on behalf of the Healthcare Information and Management Systems Society (HIMSS) and by V. Brandon Melton on behalf of the American Society for Healthcare Human Resources Administration (ASHHRA). They would like to thank all of the authors for the time and dedication that was devoted to the preparation of these chapters. The opinions expressed in this book represent the views of the individual authors and not necessarily the views of HIMSS, ASHHRA, or the American Hospital Association.

The editors would also like to thank the team of reviewers, who included Addison C. Bennett, Pacific Health Resources, Los Angeles, California; Sharon Boyce, Grossmont District Hospital, La Mesa, California; Kyle M. Gaspar, Ancilla Systems, Elk Grove Village, Illinois; Paul W. Guy, Parkview Memorial Hospital, Fort Wayne, Indiana; Frank J. Milewski, Jr., Thomas Jefferson University Hospital, Philadelphia, Pennsylvania; William J. Schwabe, Albert Einstein Medical Center, Philadelphia, Pennsylvania; Julius Spivack, Healthcare Consultant, Rochester, New York; and Mark A. Tepping, Yale-New Haven Hospital, New Haven, Connecticut.

Chapter 1

Corporate Culture: The Impact on Productivity and Performance

Francis L. Ulschak

Introduction

Take a moment and think about your current health care organization. How is it different from other health care organizations you have known of or have been associated with? For example, what are some of the differences in how work gets done? What are the attitudes toward employees and the beliefs about people? What behaviors does the health care organization reward? What behaviors are not tolerated? Who have been the heroes or heroines in your health care organization? How did they achieve that status?

Answers to these questions provide clues about the corporate culture of your health care organization. They are questions that need to be answered to determine what impact your organization's corporate culture has on its levels of performance and productivity. The thesis of this chapter is that the corporate culture of health care organizations has a direct effect on the performance and productivity of individuals and teams within these organizations.

The chapter is organized into five major sections. The first sets forth some basic assumptions about the role of corporate culture in performance and productivity.

The second section defines the concept of corporate culture. At first, this may sound like an easy thing to do. However, if you move past the popular literature and the faddish definitions, identifying what corporate culture is becomes complex. Several references are provided at the end of this chapter for readers who would like to explore the definitions and concepts of corporate culture in greater depth (Schall, 1983, p. 557; Pennings and Gresov, 1986, p. 317; Allaire and Firsirotu, 1984, p. 1983; Ouchi and Wilkins, 1985, p. 457). This chapter provides only a working definition for discussing the link between corporate culture and performance and productivity.

The third section of this chapter discusses performance and productivity at three levels—individual, team, and organization. The thesis of this section is that some aspects of corporate culture enhance performance and productivity at the individual, team, and organizational levels, and some aspects diminish performance and productivity. This section introduces the CPR + F model, which is useful for linking individual, team, and organizational performance and productivity to corporate culture.

The fourth section discusses what happens to performance and productivity when the corporate culture goes through change. Health care organizations are caught in continuous change—downsizing, merging, restructuring, and so forth. Change significantly affects the performance and productivity of individuals and teams as well as the organization as a whole.

The fifth and final section provides suggestions for assessing corporate culture. One assumption in this chapter is that certain things can be done to assess corporate culture and to intervene in ways that are desired by the health care organization. Although the degree to which corporate culture can be planned out and changed is limited, many elements of corporate culture can be controlled. Like an individual's personality, some aspects may readily be changed and other aspects will never change. However, just as it is important for the individual to know something about his or her blind side and strengths, so too is it important for the corporate culture to know something about its own strengths and weaknesses. Perhaps the primary responsibility of the health care executive today is knowing the strengths and liabilities of his or her organization's corporate culture. Only then can the executive build on the strengths and control the weaknesses.

Some Assumptions Regarding Corporate Culture

I come to this chapter with firsthand experience in downsizing a health care organization, merging two health care organizations, and building a new health care organization from scratch. These experiences, along with consultations I have been a part of and reading I have done, have led me to reach several assumptions regarding the link between corporate culture and performance and productivity.

First, *corporate cultures have a direct impact on performance and productivity.* Schein (1985, p. 24) states that individual and organizational effectiveness and the individual's feelings about the organization cannot be understood without looking at corporate culture. Desatnick (1986, p. 49), Arnold and others (1987, p. 18), Martin and Siehl (1983, p. 52), and Amsa

(1986, p. 347) all echo to various degrees the theme that corporate culture is tied closely to performance and productivity. Hence, the research indicates that health care executives who are interested in the topic of performance and productivity need to spend time considering corporate culture.

Second, *corporate culture is both a product and a process.* As a product of past experiences, corporate culture provides limits for what is possible with regard to performance and productivity. It sets boundaries because it determines how work gets done. For example, if work efficiencies come along that are contrary to corporate culture, that culture may determine that they will not be instituted. Corporate culture is a given; that is, it exists whether we want it or not.

As a process, corporate culture interacts with both the external and internal environments of the organization. This interaction brings about changes in the corporate culture. Hence, corporate culture is not only a given; it is also flexible. It changes over the life cycle of an organization.

Adizes (1979, p. 3) provides an excellent model that links the life cycle of an organization to its corporate culture. According to this model, the corporate culture needed in the start-up phase of an organization is characterized by intense action and quick decisions, whereas later in the life cycle of the organization, more strategic planning and administrative functions are needed.

Because corporate culture changes along with the environment in which it finds itself, decision makers can plan for their corporate culture and, to some degree, create it according to their own intentions. My recent experience in the start-up phase of an organization is one of intentional corporate culture building. We continuously asked these questions: What corporate culture do we want to build? How are the decisions we are making in line with that corporate culture? Are we investing our resources in those things that further that corporate culture?

The third assumption is that *corporate culture is visible and tangible.* Think about your initial reactions to health care organizations you have joined or visited. Remember the different feelings you had. Some were warm and friendly. Others were businesslike. Remember how the organizations were visibly different. Think about the way the offices were decorated and how they looked.

I believe that one reason guest relations are so critical in health care organizations today is because decision makers are becoming more concerned about the feelings their organizations generate. They know that in a competitive market, patients and their families are particularly sensitive to corporate culture. The message that health care organizations want to send is that they value their patients, their families, and their employees.

Fourth, *no one corporate culture is best for a health care organization.* The question is not what is the best corporate culture, but how is the current corporate culture working? Is it effective in getting the work of the health care organization done? If not, what is getting in the way? What elements of the corporate culture need to be changed, kept the same, or added? Corporate culture needs to be viewed in light of how to build on strengths and how to identify and control for limitations.

Barney (1986, p. 656) has an excellent discussion of the problems of trying to duplicate the corporate culture of another organization. His main point is that successful corporate cultures are the products of their own unique conditions and cannot be imitated without introducing flaws. If they were easy to imitate, everyone would do it, and the successful corporate culture would no longer have a competitive edge. The challenge Barney poses for persons interested in corporate culture is not to try to imitate a successful corporate culture but to understand their own unique corporate culture.

Fifth, *not all corporate cultures are equally effective.* Although no one corporate culture is ideal, the reality is that some corporate cultures are going to be more effective than others. Block (1987, p. 20) discusses two cultural mind-sets in organizations: the bureaucratic and the entrepreneurial. The bureaucratic mind-set has characteristics such as top-down management, occasional emphasis on employee self-interest to the exclusion of the interests of the organization as a whole, dependency of employees on the organization, and a general belief that the way to get ahead is through manipulating the system. The entrepreneurial mind-set has characteristics such as emphasis on employees' taking responsibility for their roles and actions, enlightened self-interest (that is, having employee self-interest that aligns with organizationwide interests), authentic management that deals directly and truthfully with issues and problems, and an expectation of autonomous behavior on the part of the employees.

Certain elements position an organization for success with regard to performance and productivity. These elements include (1) individual and team commitment to tasks, (2) clarity of purpose and role at individual and team levels, and (3) systems for providing individuals and teams with feedback on how they are doing. Corporate culture needs to support each of these elements.

Sixth, *being aware of corporate culture is good business.* Many times, those who work in the human resources departments of health care organizations are perceived as the only ones who are concerned about corporate culture. But corporate culture affects all aspects of the health care organization—direct patient care, revenue-producing departments, and the business office—not just the human resources department. It is a mistake for staff members at every level to regard corporate culture as the responsibility of the human resources department. Corporate culture defines how work will get done. It defines what performance and productivity will be. Sister Regina Clifton (1986, p. 50) has stated: "Maintaining a religious organization's corporate culture is as essential to its survival as meeting the budget, developing a strategic plan, or recruiting physicians; if one is not serious about undertaking that responsibility, he or she should look for a new job."

These are some of the assumptions I have regarding corporate culture. I have included numerous references in this chapter as an invitation for further reading. I encourage you to develop your own set of assumptions so that you have a model for understanding and working with the corporate culture of your organization.

Corporate Culture: What Is It?

Before we define corporate culture, think for a moment about the following two organizations and your feelings toward each:

- **Organization A:** The *structure* of Organization A is flat; few layers exist between the first-line supervisor and top-level management. The organization is set up to work from a matrix design, which means that when new projects come along, project teams, task forces, or both are formed.

  Decision making is done quickly and efficiently. The chief executive officer makes many decisions on the spot. The general operating norm is that the organization cannot wait for a long decision-making process. Decision making may happen in informal ways, that is, in hallways and informal discussions or in formal meetings using formal processes.

  The organization's *view of managers* is that managers are major assets to the organization. The organization spends a significant amount of money on management recruitment, selection, development, training, and compensation. Managers are hired because of their success as cutting-edge managers in their previous positions, and they are expected to continue to be cutting-edge managers in their areas. Managers are decision makers; the general operating principle is that it is easier to ask for forgiveness than for permission.

  Compensation is built around the merit system. Individuals are compensated for meeting objectives and standards. Some team incentives are included for work on project teams and task forces.

  Patients are important to Organization A, which has a strong service emphasis. Patient information is aggressively sought. The organization is constantly monitoring patient feedback and takes that feedback to the highest levels of the organization. Patients are seen as the customers, and every effort is made to ensure as pleasant a stay as possible for the patients and their families.
- **Organization B:** The *structure* of Organization B is hierarchical. With three to four layers between the first-line supervisor and the chief executive officer, emphasis is on following the chain of command. In discussions of new projects, participants must always determine whose area of responsibility would cover such projects.

  Decision making is made at the highest levels, with an emphasis on lengthy processes designed to ensure the right decision. If new items come up, they need to wait until the start of the decision-making process, for example, the beginning of the next fiscal year. Responsiveness is slow but methodical.

The organization's *view of managers* is that managers should be rewarded for following the system. Many of them have grown up in the system and have learned to follow the rules closely. Conservative actions are encouraged. The key operating principle is to keep upper management informed of every move and to minimize responsibility for mistakes.

Compensation is made partly on the basis of merit but mainly on the basis of longevity. Longtime service and loyalty to the health care organization are of primary importance.

The general attitude toward *patients* is: "Patients come to us. We are the ones who know health care. They need to trust in us and the years of service we have in the community." Only a few questions are asked regarding the patients' experiences with the health care organization.

Organizations A and B represent two very different corporate cultures. Having read about them, ask yourself these questions: How would it feel for you to be part of Organization A? Organization B? Which organization would you prefer to work with?

Neither organization has the right corporate culture; rather, each has a corporate culture with its own unique flavor. The effectiveness of each organization depends on how the culture matches the expectations of the marketplace in which it finds itself.

Corporate culture is essentially the set of assumptions that health care organizations make about people, how people work together, and the best way to get work done. Schein (1985, p. 9) writes that corporate culture is:

A pattern of basic assumptions—invented, discovered, or developed by a given group as it learns to cope with its problems of external adaptation and internal integration—that has worked well enough to be considered valid and therefore, to be taught to new members as the correct way to perceive, think and feel in relation to those problems.

Schein's definition has several important parts. First, *corporate culture is a pattern of basic assumptions.* It is not simplistic; rather, it is like a finely woven garment with intricate patterns. A corollary is that corporate culture is not easily described. Some cultural norms, such as those concerning dress and appearance, can be easily observed, but the deeper aspects of corporate culture, such as norms about the management of conflict among the organization's members, are not readily apparent. Determining an organization's culture cannot be done by simply passing around a questionnaire or making quick observations, which only result in superficial data. Like anthropologists who spend years living in a culture and observing it before the deeper assumptions are discovered, persons studying corporate culture need to commit themselves to a long and methodical process.

Another corollary is that not all aspects of corporate culture are equally important. Although some aspects of a culture are interesting but unimportant, other aspects are vital links in the foundation of the culture. This becomes very important when steps are taken to alter the corporate culture.

The second important part of Schein's definition is that *corporate culture is invented, discovered, or developed by a given group as it learns to cope with its problems of external adaptation and internal integration.* In other words, corporate culture is learned as the organization grows and develops. The members of the organization learn what works, what makes the organization successful, and how it can survive in the world. To understand how corporate culture is learned, people must have an understanding of organizational growth cycles and critical events in the life of an organization. Each critical event is a time of testing the basic assumptions. Will the basic assumptions continue to work? Will they still be useful? Will the organization still survive?

Sometimes, workers in a corporate culture do not know the reasons for behaving in a certain way. A common attitude is "We do it this way because we have always done it," which betrays a certain "amnesia" in the corporate culture that makes it difficult to change. The typical member of the organization is not fully aware that some of the assumptions of the culture are working against his or her attempts at creativity and innovation.

The presence of amnesia in a corporate culture is akin to the story of the preparation of the Thanksgiving Day ham. As the father of the family is preparing the ham for Thanksgiving dinner, he cuts both ends off the ham. When someone asks him why, he says that the ham "breathes" better this way and, consequently, it cooks better. Besides, his father always did it this way. So the inquirer goes to the father's father and asks him why he cut the ends off the ham. The response is the same: "So the ham can breathe better. And my father always did it that way." But when the inquirer goes to the father's father's father and asks him about the ham, his response is different: "I cut both ends off because the pan was too small." Once enshrined, the reasons why something is done may no longer be clear—you do it because that is the way it is done. And the rationale for it is made up as time goes along.

The third important part of Schein's definition is that *the pattern of basic assumptions has worked sufficiently well to be taught to new members as the way in which work should be done.* The members of the organization believe so strongly in the ways they get work done that they believe the new members need to be taught those same ways. A key part of orienting new members to the organization is teaching them the basic assumptions. Part of new member acculturation is hearing statements like "this is how we do things here" and "this is the way we have been successful in the past." Orientation programs such as those conducted at Walt Disney World are designed to teach cultural expectations and to entice employees to "buy into" those expectations. In an organization that is aware of its culture and values, the recruitment, selection, orientation, and training processes will be focused not only on the technical skills but also on the cultural fit.

When a health care organization is faced with change, basic assumptions about how to do business are called into question. For example, the way of doing business for many hospitals has changed in the past five years because of the introduction of the prospective pricing system. The basic assumptions were found to be lacking. The old assumptions were no longer "useful" and, in fact, no longer supported hospital survival. It was only when an outsider came along and asked "why do you do it that way?" that hospitals even thought about their assumptions for doing business.

The basic assumptions comprising corporate culture affect the total business enterprise. The next section will focus on the impact of corporate culture on performance and productivity at the individual, team, and organizational levels.

Effects of Corporate Culture on Productivity and Performance

Corporate culture affects the performance and productivity of individuals, teams, and the organization as a whole. The purpose of this section is to discuss the effects of corporate culture and provide a model for viewing the relationship between corporate culture and performance and productivity. That model, the CPR + F model, is illustrated in figure 1-1.

In health care organizations, performance and productivity are products of people investing themselves in an organization. Consequently, the key

Figure 1-1.   The CPR + F Model

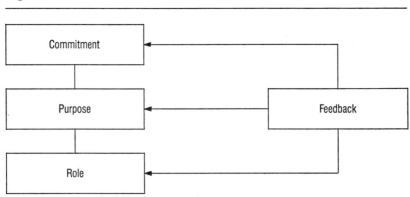

questions to be addressed are: What is it that causes people to invest themselves in an organization? What is it that takes an "average performer" and makes him or her an "outstanding performer"? What is it that causes a person to work long hours until a project is completed? The answer is *commitment,* the first part of the CPR + F model. Commitment is what turns performance from average to outstanding. It is commitment that causes individuals to put in extra hours, live through the frustration of roadblocks, and put up with working conditions that other persons might not put up with.

Purpose is the second part of the model. Individuals feel a strong sense of purpose when they understand what it is they are contributing to the corporate venture. That strong sense of purpose is also felt when the contributions of individuals are valued by both the individuals themselves and by the organization they serve.

The third part of the CPR + F model is *role,* or how individuals express their commitment and purpose in the organization. Their role is how they go about their work and how they cooperate with others.

Feedback, the fourth part, is providing employees with information on how they are doing. Individuals need to receive feedback with regard to commitment, purpose, and role.

The CPR + F model suggests that when commitment is high, purpose and role are clear. It also suggests that when feedback loops are present between all three, the performance and productivity of individuals is high. If confusion exists in any of these elements, the other three elements are diminished, and performance and productivity drop. Corporate culture can strengthen or weaken any part of the CPR + F model as it applies to the individual employee, a team of employees, or the organization as a whole.

Individual Productivity and Performance

The individual is the basic building block of the team and the organization. If the individual "buys into" or "enrolls" in the mission of the team and the organization, the result is a committed individual who helps the team and the organization attain high performance and productivity.

Commitment

Think about an organization that you were highly committed to. What was happening in the organization? What was it that invited your commitment? What was it that got you to personally invest in the organization? Now think about an organization that you have been part of but did not invest in. What was happening in that organization? If you were to summarize your answers to these questions, what would you say?

The question of how to increase commitment can be approached in many ways. I have found that individuals invest in their employers when they see the linkage between what the organization is asking of them and their own need fulfillment. They invest when there is a sense that the team or organization is fulfilling important needs that they have.

On the surface, the process of increasing commitment might be like the classic behavioral model of stimulus and response. The model looks like this:

Stimulus⟶ Response

The organization offers a stimulus and the individual provides a response. The organization provides an across-the-board salary increase (stimulus) and the individual feels rewarded (response).

However, this classic model is misleading because it does not take into account what is really happening, which looks like this:

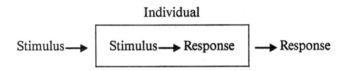

The organization provides a stimulus that goes into the individual's internal world. The individual evaluates the stimulus in light of core needs and on the basis of this internal stimulus and response makes an external response. In the previous example, the salary increase is designed to make the individual feel rewarded. However, if in the internal world of the individual he or she is already feeling salary injustice, the reward may increase dissatisfaction. The critical aspect of this revised model is that in order to understand commitment, you need to get inside the individual and understand his or her internal stimulus and response. That internal stimulus and response has to do with need fulfillment.

What are the core needs that need to be considered? Other authors have their own lists of core needs, and so the following list is not to be seen as exclusive. Nevertheless, it is a list that I have found important to consider. The core needs that affect the stimulus-response process are (1) accomplishment and recognition, (2) structure and control, (3) social relations, and (4) creativity and playfulness.

Accomplishment and recognition are key experiences that encourage individuals to invest in the organization. To be able to feel internal fulfillment of a job well done and to have external recognition for it are major stimuli for even higher performance and productivity. Recently, I had a discussion with a hospital engineer and asked him what was rewarding in his job. He suggested that we walk down the hallways of the hospital and see the completed projects. As we walked, he pointed out to me the projects that he had done. Accomplishment and recognition are cornerstones of investment.

Structure and control are another core need for all individuals. Probably the most feared experience is that of losing control. Behind the usual lists of most fear-provoking events, for example, public speaking, is the fear that a person will lose control of himself or herself or of the setting. Structure is what gives a person a sense of predictability and of being in control. Structure provides the channels for a person's energy and prevents anarchy. Individuals need a sense of structure and control to make sense of the events about them.

Social relations are a core need fulfilled by a person's work life. Working people spend many of their waking hours at work. For many employees, work is not only a place to make money but to make friends and have a social life. That is why some individuals refuse to take a promotion and leave their work unit. That is also why what appears to be a small organizational restructuring takes on such importance to some individuals. What the organization regards as a restructuring is for these persons a major shifting of their social ties. Organizations can address the need for social relations by encouraging team building and informal get-togethers such as sports events or quality circles.

Creativity and playfulness are another core need. All individuals need to experience creativity. The frequent source of that creativity is playfulness. I like to use the word *plurking* to identify appropriate mixtures of working and playing. *Plurking* is combining the attitude of playfulness with work accomplishment. The result is an individual who stays energized at work. A playful attitude at work provides the energies for high levels of creativity and for the work to get done.

Recently, I discussed *plurking* with an individual from Apple Computer. In turn, she asked me, "Do you know the difference between a Boy Scout troop and a group of Apple Computer employees?" I responded with a "no" and she said, "The Boy Scouts have adult leadership!" Now, that is an example of playfulness brought into the work setting.

All individuals bring these needs and others into the workplace. In the past, a misconception was that individual needs are to be kept out of the workplace. When an individual walked in the door of the health care organization, all individual needs were left outside. First of all, we now know that is impossible to do. We are whole human beings, and as such we bring all that we are to work. Second, it is the need-fulfillment or feeling side of individuals that has the energy. If we want invested, turned-on individuals, we need to address and invite them to expect need fulfillment at work. The degree to which these needs are met furthers the commitment of individuals to their organizations.

What is important is that commitment is a feeling. If an organization is looking for committed individuals, it needs to be open to expressions of feelings and fully functioning human beings. Organizations looking for high levels of performance and productivity in their employees need to build a corporate culture that is supportive of the expression of feelings and the fulfillment of individual needs as well as organizational needs.

Decision makers who are studying corporate culture must realize, however, that commitment is subject to rapid changes. Managers who neglect giving their employees a clear sense of purpose soon find that employee commitment weakens. But individuals who lose a sense of commitment can readily make another commitment given the proper conditions, such as when managers show them once again how their needs can be met.

Purpose

The question now becomes: committed to what? Commitment is not a general condition; it is tied to something. An individual cannot be committed to nothing. A clear sense of purpose is needed. But purpose is in the eyes of the individual. The individual needs to know what the purpose is.

Perhaps one of the most powerful descriptions of the role of purpose is in Frankl's (1963) *Man's Search for Meaning*. Frankl describes the power of purpose and meaning in the intolerable conditions of a concentration camp during World War II. His observations were that people in that setting who had meaning and could sense a purpose in the experience were the survivors. But those who lost purpose and meaning quickly succumbed to the conditions.

Countless examples can be found of people with a clear sense of purpose taking on all kinds of odds and coming out victorious. One example is the dedication and purpose of the founders of MADD (Mothers against Drunk Driving), who began a movement that is now a powerful, nationwide organization. They had a purpose and were committed to it.

The same success can be brought to the workplace if an organization gives its employees a clear sense of purpose. But the organization also has to find out whether the employees are buying into that purpose and how their work lives are changing as a result. If an employee cannot accept all of the parts of a statement of purpose, the organization needs to identify which parts are unacceptable and address them.

When employees have a sense of purpose that what they are doing makes a difference, phenomenal energies get released. When those energies get channeled into work, the result is outstanding performance and productivity. The implication for the organization is that it needs to discuss purpose with employees, sell it to them, and orient their work lives toward it. The organization needs to understand that the key is not just the organization's saying "here is the purpose." Rather, the organization must spend time to help the individual tie into the organization's purpose. The organization needs to be "employee centered" if it is to fully tap the individual's commitment and energy.

There is a classic line from a John Belushi and Dan Aykroyd movie, "The Blues Brothers." These two very unlikely brothers, recently out of jail, are asked what it is that they are doing and the response is: "We are on a mission from God." It is interesting to imagine what would happen if the employees in our health care organizations went about their work with that sense of purpose, for purpose is a powerful invitation to investment.

Role

The third part of the CPR + F model as it applies to individuals is that of role clarity. Role clarity means that individuals understand and agree with what their roles are and understand their relationships with other workers. They understand and agree with how they are to fulfill their purpose in the organization.

Pareek (1980, p. 143) talks about the concept of role efficacy. Efficacy is the potential effectiveness of how the role gets lived out. It involves questions such as: Does the individual feel valued by the organization? Is the role a central one to getting the work done? If role efficacy is strong, the individual has a sense of being a major contributor to the organization and understands the link to other employees.

Feedback

Thus far, we have discussed the foundation elements of the CPR + F model as it applies to the individual. We have clues about how commitment, purpose, and role are linked to corporate culture. However, how do we keep those three elements alive and relevant to the needs of the organization? How do we deal with changing levels of commitment or changing roles? The answer is to implement feedback systems.

Each individual needs to get feedback on his or her commitment, purpose, and role. Feedback is a mechanism to correct for the inevitable changes in the organization. Like a fancy, high-performance automobile with a multitude of gauges designed to keep the driver informed of the running condition, feedback systems let individuals know whether they are winning or out of sync with their role, purpose, or commitment. Examples of feedback mechanisms are performance reviews, questionnaires, staff meetings, and interviews.

The Organization's Response to the Individual Worker

The CPR + F model suggests that high performance and productivity are a result of (1) individuals who have a strong commitment and a clear sense of purpose and role and (2) feedback systems that provide individuals with good data. Hence, the corporate culture of an organization needs to enhance and support all four parts of the CPR + F model.

First, the corporate culture needs to be clear about the organization's purpose and mission. For example, in my setting, everyone who comes through orientation hears one message: "We are in the business of fighting cancer through patient care, education, and research." Regardless of where the person may work, there is one profoundly simple message, and it is a message that the individual can commit to.

The corporate culture needs to ensure that its purpose is communicated not only during orientation of new employees but also during the employee recruitment and selection process, as well as during orientation updates and in internal publications and statements made by the chief executive officer. The corporate culture needs to value communicating the purpose and to invest energy in ongoing communications. There can never be too much communication about purpose. The error most organizations make is assuming that talking about its purpose once or putting it in an organizational publication is sufficient. The danger exists for an organization's purpose to become muddy, especially during changing times. Hence, the corporate culture needs to support ongoing discussions.

The second organizational response is that corporate culture needs to invite commitment by auditing the ways in which individual and organizational purpose can stay in line. In part, this means engaging individuals in discussions about how an organization's purpose fits with an individual's purpose. The corporate culture needs to be sensitive to individual needs and to how core needs get fulfilled in the workplace. When an individual believes that it is his or her product, not the organization's, both the organization and the individual win.

The third response is that corporate culture needs to clarify the roles of its employees. Although role conflict is inevitable in the changing world of health care, the corporate culture needs to value conflict management or role renegotiation (Sherwood and Glidewell, 1973, p. 195). Role renegotiation is a process by which individuals and the organization identify initial role expectations and then monitor those roles to see when role expectations begin to shift. A major assumption of role renegotiation is that role shifts will happen and that performance and productivity will drop off as a result. Therefore, it behooves the organization to (1) encourage individuals to feel comfortable about pointing out role "pinches" and (2) renegotiate roles with individuals as necessary.

Finally, corporate culture needs to value and facilitate feedback to the individual on his or her commitment, purpose, and role. The bottom line is that the outstanding performer is the individual who is committed, who has a clear idea of purpose and role, and who is receiving feedback from his or her employer.

Team Productivity and Performance

Although most organizations are dependent on teams of people to get the work done, this is especially true for health care organizations, which are labor intensive and are by nature interdependent. Patient care involves teams that include doctors, nurses, laboratory technicians, pharmacists, and others who work together to deliver the product of good care. Health care organizations that are built around the "lone ranger" principle are unique and are not likely to survive.

Teams are groups of people who are dependent on one another to get work done. They have common objectives and have a shared accountability for completing their tasks. Teams are sometimes formed across departments and sometimes within a department.

As with individuals, corporate culture has a major influence on the performance and productivity of a team because it provides boundaries for that performance and productivity. In other words, it defines how the work will get done. One way to describe the link between corporate culture and effective teams is to use the CPR + F model.

Commitment

Effective teams have high levels of commitment to the team itself and to the members of the team. A team without high levels of commitment is not achieving its potential for high productivity and performance. If the members of the team are not committed, the result is a drop-off of team performance. It is like playing basketball with one member of the team playing half-court; the rest of the team can carry the person for awhile but not for long. Eventually, the team gets tired and begins to resent the half-court player.

Frequently, when I am working with teams, I ask them the following questions: "On a 10-point scale, how committed are you to this team?" "Also on a 10-point scale, how committed do you think the others are to this team?" Many times, team members tell me that no one has ever before asked them about their level of commitment, and yet commitment is vital to their functioning.

What does it take for a team to be committed? Many of the comments that were made in reference to individuals also apply here. The crucial element is that the members of the team perceive that their needs are getting met by being part of the team. Jones and Bearley (1986, p. 10) provide a law of commitment that says: "Meaningful participation leads to a sense of involvement that evokes a feeling of influence that generates psychological ownership that results in commitment."

The necessary ingredient is that the individual perceives that his or her participation is meaningful. This is important to note when considering participative management. If the manager using participative decision making does not really value the individual's input or is really using it as a way of selling decisions already made, the result is a decrease of commitment on he part of the team members. People need to perceive that their participation is meaningful.

Within teams in large organizations, commitment and loyalty are frequently directed toward the team, not toward the organization. The organization is distant—it is something out there. But the team is real because its members spend eight hours a day working in it. In this case, loyalties to the organization are spin-offs of loyalty to the team.

Purpose

The purpose of the team needs to be clear to each of the team members. They need to know their purpose for being together so that they can align themselves accordingly. They need to know what the outcomes are and what winning means. And they need a vision of what they can really be or become.

As with the individual, the team's purpose needs to be in line with the organization's purpose. This is crucial with teams because they have their own corporate culture. That corporate culture can have three orientations (Martin and Siehl, 1983, p. 52):

- It can enhance the organization's corporate culture; that is, it can have the same values and purpose. This is the team that managers want to manage. The team is in line with and focused on the organization.
- It can be "orthogonal" to the organization's corporate culture; that is, it can have a value system and purpose that differ from those of the organization but do not detract from the organization. The business office in a health care setting may be orthogonal. The work of the business office has its own set of principles and values that may not be the same as the overall corporate culture but is not opposed to it.
- It can be a corporate counterculture; that is, it can have values and purposes that are at odds with the organization. This is the team that managers dread. Team members, at best, are open with their hostility toward organizational practices and, at worst, work underground to subvert the organization's policies. Bates (1984, p. 43) provides examples of corporate countercultures and how they block the work of the organization. He provides an example of how organizational corporate culture can act as a block to change and to problem resolution.

An exercise that I have found useful in working with teams and assisting them in developing purpose statements is Block's vision of greatness (1987, p. 99). The process first involves the team's envisioning what it would be like to be a "great team." This causes the team to think outside of its normal boundaries of thinking. Then, the exercise asks the team to define a vision of greatness with regard to purpose, commitment, and roles:

- Purpose: What would the team look like and how would it behave if it had a vision of greatness with regard to its purpose?
- Commitment: What behaviors would be present in a team that had a vision of greatness with regard to the commitment of each of its members to the team and to the organization as a whole?
- Roles: What behaviors would be present if there were a vision of greatness with regard to roles?

Other areas for formulating vision-of-greatness statements can include vision of greatness regarding relationships with users, clients, or customers; vision of greatness in team-member relations; and vision of greatness in the production of services or products. Once the team members decide what greatness means for them as a team, they have defined an ideal future that they collectively desire and can move toward.

Role

Because team members are interdependent — no one person can do the job alone — the role of each member must be clear to everyone. Hence, it is important for the organization to engage in role negotiation and have renegotiation systems in place. Members of the team need an appreciation for their dependency on one another.

I sometimes use an exercise that asks all the team members sitting around a table to share how they are dependent on each other. Each member of the team shares how it is that he or she is dependent on every person on the team. Once the exercise is completed, the team has an open discussion about how negotiated dependency is healthy and, indeed, vital to health care organizations.

Feedback

Feedback is the "breakfast of champions." Like individuals, teams need feedback on how they are doing in order to strengthen their commitment, their sense of purpose, and the effectiveness of their roles. Some methods of feedback include regular meetings, questionnaires, and interviews.

The Organization's Response to Its Teams

Every health care organization needs to strengthen the commitment, clarity of purpose, and clarity of roles of each of its teams. Three steps can be taken:

- The corporate culture needs to identify norms, or accepted patterns of behavior among individuals, which endorse and support teams and clarify their commitment and purpose.
- The corporate culture needs to encourage problem-solving, conflict management, and decision-making skills as they apply to teams.
- The corporate culture needs to have structures in place for rewarding team accomplishment. High levels of team performance and productivity cannot be attained if the reward system still only recognizes individual performance and productivity. Teams have to have reward systems directed toward them as well.

Teams are a powerful force in the performance and productivity of an organization. The organization has a choice — either manage the development, training, performance, and productivity of teams or ignore them and let them develop on their own. Teams will always be an integral part of health care organizations. Decision makers must decide whether the corporate culture is managing them.

Organizational Productivity and Performance

Thus far, we have discussed individual and team performance and productivity and have shown how they are linked to corporate culture. An effective corporate culture encourages individual and team commitment, ensures clarity of purpose and roles, and uses feedback systems. The true power of the organization is released when there is congruity between individual, team, and organizational commitment, purpose, and role.

The purpose of this section is to identify the factors that contribute to high performance and productivity at the organizational level. Adizes (1979, pp. 5–7) identifies four managerial functions that are essential:

- *Productive:* The organization needs to produce services and products. This is stating the obvious; the reason an organization comes into existence is to produce a service or product.
- *Administrative:* The organization needs to have policies and procedures that define the way things get done.
- *Entrepreneurial:* The organization needs creativity and innovation to continue its existence.
- *Integrative:* The organization needs mechanisms for bringing the work of individuals and teams together. Organizations are formed because a single person cannot do the work. When numerous individuals and teams are involved, efforts need to be integrated.

For the organization to be in its prime, that is, the place of greatest organizational productivity and performance, it needs all four of these functions in place. The most critical function that keeps the organization in its prime is the entrepreneurial (E) function. The message for health care organizations is that the E function is vital to maintaining a growing organization. This is especially true in a changing environment.

The four managerial functions of an organization need to be nurtured by the corporate culture if these functions are to grow. As we have seen, corporate culture represents the core assumptions of the organization. Behind these assumptions are the fundamental values of an organization. These values drive the organization and the goals and objectives that grow from this core of values (figure 1-2). The structures of the organization are in turn determined by the values, goals, and objectives ("form follows function"). It is important that the organization examine its goals, objectives, and structures to see that they are in line with the desired corporate culture.

Figure 1-2. Relationship of Values to an Organization's Corporate Culture

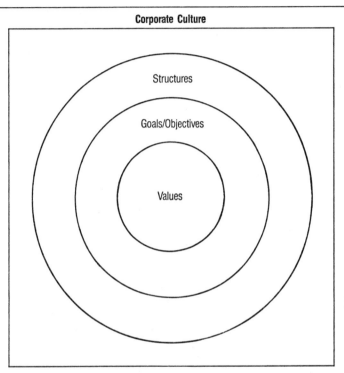

Corporate Culture

Structures

Goals/Objectives

Values

Corporate Culture and Change

When the corporate culture is oriented toward high performance and productivity, a harmony exists between the values, goals, objectives, and structures of the organization, and these are in sync with the commitment, purpose, and roles of the individuals and teams of the organization. However, internal positioning for high performance and productivity is not enough. If the organization has not stayed in sync with the external environment, the internal positioning will mean nothing. The cosmic joke is that an organization may have carefully positioned itself internally but may have nowhere to go because the markets have shifted. No corporate culture can compensate for a lack of market. Consequently, decision makers must monitor change.

Change is a given in health care organizations. Think about your experiences in health care in the past five years. What have been the changes in your experience? Some that stand out for me are changing demographics, an older population, growing self-help movements, shifting reimbursement patterns, nursing shortages, competition for markets, and a growing number of ambulatory care centers. In the years ahead, the ability of supercomputers to handle huge volumes of information in more sophisticated ways will have a major impact on health care institutions. Those supercomputers will provide us with information in ways that would astound us today. The list of changes, both past and present, could go on and on.

Think about one of those changes — shifting reimbursement patterns — which has had a major effect on the business of health care organizations. Many of these organizations have found that their corporate culture — the assumptions that were successful in the past — now no longer work. Some organizations have changed, some have gone out of business, and some have prospered. I believe that an organizational culture that permits flexibility and change is an important factor in the organization's survival.

When an organization makes any significant change — whether that change is restructuring, merging, downsizing, or starting a new business — the immediate result is a drop in performance and productivity. Changes cause uncertainty with regard to commitment, purpose, and role for the individual, team, and organization. Even if the change is a restructuring that appears to clarify a perceived problem, the immediate result is a drop in performance and productivity, because individuals need time to internalize their new commitment, role, or purpose. Time that was previously spent productively is now spent trying to figure out what the new purpose or role is. Change in an organization is like surgery: if it is significant, it takes the patient awhile to recover.

The important ingredient for a successful corporate culture is the degree to which the corporate culture has built-in assumptions that allow for change and flexibility. If the corporate culture is rigid and unchanging, changes are difficult to make, and if the environment is turbulent, the organization likely cannot survive. If the corporate culture has assumptions built into it that allow for change, such as those arising from the CPR + F model, the organization may grow and prosper in a time of rapid change.

Assessment of Corporate Culture

Thus far, this chapter has been concerned with corporate culture and how it affects performance and productivity. Now the questions are: How do we assess corporate culture? If corporate culture can potentially limit performance and productivity at the levels of the individual, team, and organization, how do we begin to change that? How do we identify the aspects of corporate culture that work for us and those that work against us?

Three important points must be made before we can begin to answer these questions. The first point is that there are many layers of corporate culture. The iceberg model in figure 1-3 illustrates this concept. At the surface level, corporate culture is known by the way employees dress, the way the building is decorated, the stories that are told about the successes and the failures of the enterprise, and so forth. This information is easy to get

Figure 1-3. The Iceberg Model of Corporate Culture

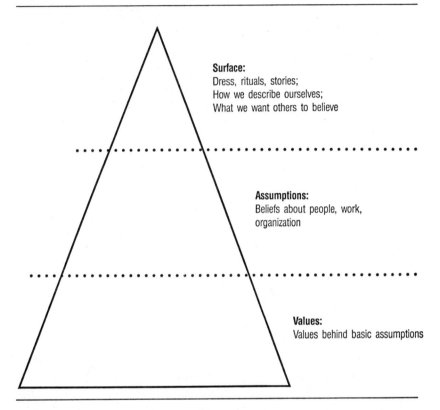

during an assessment. However, the real work of determining a corporate culture is below the surface. Here lie the critical values and assumptions regarding the corporate culture. These values and assumptions are more difficult to determine.

Second, just as a change in an individual's behavior sometimes results in a significant change in his or her attitude and self-concept, so too does a change in the observable behaviors within the organization sometimes result in changes in the values and assumptions. For example, staff improvements in guest relations may change surface behaviors and also begin to affect the basic assumptions and underlying values of the corporate culture. Patients would not only be treated as guests but would start being *regarded* as guests by new and seasoned employees alike.

Third, there are three times when employees are most sensitive to corporate culture:

- *When they enter the organization:* When people first enter the organization, they are most sensitive to the corporate culture. I like to ask

people who join my department to provide me with comments about the things that they find different in this organization. That is the beginning of their understanding of our culture.
- *When they leave the organization:* Exit interviews can be a time when the deeper levels of corporate culture are uncovered. As people leave the organization, they once again take off their blinders to the organization and can provide insights into the culture.
- *When there are major disruptions in the organization:* During times of crisis, people have a certain distance from the organization that allows them to talk about it. In addition, the crises themselves identify what is critical for the organization. These are ideal times to identify what is happening with corporate culture.

A number of assessment strategies are available in the literature (Reynierse and Harker, 1986, p. 1; Flexner and Gunkler, 1986, p. 38; Gross and Shichman, 1987, p. 52; Atchison, 1988, p. 15). Some are simple, and some are complex. Some deal with the surface elements of corporate culture; some go for the in-depth aspects of culture. Each provides a step toward the identification of corporate culture.

The process suggested here is built on the assumptions that were identified earlier in this chapter. First, not all of corporate culture is knowable. Second, not all aspects of corporate culture are equally important (some of the surface aspects really do not matter during assessments of corporate culture). Third, the key to a successful assessment is not the identification of the perfect corporate culture but rather the discovery of the current corporate culture.

The goal of the assessment is to understand the values and assumptions of the corporate culture that are affecting individual and team commitment, clarity of purpose, and clarity of role, as well as the effectiveness of the feedback systems. Once the values and assumptions are understood, decision makers can ask the question: What, if anything, do we need to be changing, adding, or subtracting?

Step 1: Identification of What Is

The first step is understanding what the corporate culture currently is. In addition to looking at the components of the CPR + F model, this includes conducting an audit of the internal human resource functions and an assessment of the messages being sent via recruitment, selection, orientation, training, compensation, and benefits programs, as well as via promotion strategies, job design, and employee assistance programs.

Data collection can be done in a number of ways. Ulschak (1983) provides a discussion of a number of standard assessment strategies:

- *Observations:* How does the organization get its work done? Where and how is commitment evident in the workplace? What is the level of commitment? To what degree do individuals and teams act with a sense of purpose? How is an understanding of and agreement with the organization's purpose evident? Do individuals and teams demonstrate clarity of roles? How? When role conflicts occur, what happens to the individuals involved? What tone is felt in the organization?

- *Questionnaires:* A number of questionnaires focus on corporate culture directly or indirectly. Some of the sources cited in this chapter present established questionnaires (Arnold and others, 1987; Atchison, 1988; Desatnick, 1986; Reynierse, 1986). The questions are designed to determine the individual's sense of alignment with the organization in terms of commitment, purpose, and roles, as well as to determine the effectiveness of feedback systems. Questions asked of employees include: Do you understand the mission of the organization? Are you committed to that mission? What are the values that you see at the core of this organization? Do your values align themselves with those core values? Do you understand your role in the organization? Does the organization understand your role?

- *Print media:* Print media refers to what an organization says about itself in promotional material, interviews with executives, and internal communication tools (newsletters, journals, and so forth). This rich source of data can be tapped in ways that are unobtrusive; that is, you do not have to take people away from their work. As you go through the print media, ask yourself these questions: How is the organization presenting itself? What message does it want to communicate? What aspects of the organization are emphasized? Do the organization's purpose and mission come across in a clear way? What values are behind the stories and pictures?

- *Interviews:* Along with questionnaires, interviewing is one of the most common methods of assessing corporate culture, and for me, it is the most interesting. Ask employees about the culture. What are the rituals that are important in the organization? For example, what is it that the organization puts forward in a significant way? (The budget process? Performance review? Employee recognition?) What are the stories around the organization with regard to successes? Who are the successful employees of the past and present? What are the stories about failure? What are the mission and purpose of the organization, and are they understood? How do employee values match those of the organization? What is it that employees are committed to in this organization? How valued is each employee and his or her role? The potential questions continue on indefinitely. Interviews allow you to go after in-depth information and explore employees' perceptions in detail.

- *Focus groups:* External audiences such as key suppliers and client groups can be invited to participate in focus groups that reveal how they see the health care organization. These external audiences may be picking up subtle messages that the organization is sending but that the organization may not even be aware of. In particular, focus groups are sources of data regarding how commitment, clarity of purpose and roles, and feedback mechanisms are perceived by the community at large. Marketing surveys often use focus groups to obtain such data.

- *Internal and external combination:* Identification of corporate culture is a humbling experience because you are trying to become aware of something that you are also part of. That is why it is useful to use external resources in combination with internal resources. Schein (1985, p. 112) suggests that the ideal combination is one that pairs an external person with an internal person. The external person spends some time wandering around the organization and gathering observations. When the time comes to meet with the internal person, the external person brings the element of newness and surprise to the conversation. He or she will say, "Why is it done that way?" The internal person brings the experience of the organization and provides the data. Between the two, corporate culture can begin to be sorted out. Eventually, the pair meets with other people in the organization to discuss their findings.

Because all of the preceding methods have strengths and weaknesses, I find it useful to use two or three methods. If there is a "triangulation," that is, if two or more sources of data are pointing in the same direction, you can be more certain that you are on the right track. But keep in mind that the methods I am suggesting are generic. Use what fits.

With the advent of widespread interest in corporate culture, interest in buying cultural assessment tools from consultants has also become widespread. Such tools should be approached cautiously. For some consultants, the development of their cultural assessment tool was simply a renaming of their client survey, attitude survey, management style survey, or some other tool. Although some of these tools begin to assess corporate culture, no single questionnaire can identify much more than the surface elements. Questionnaires that promise you an in-depth cultural examination and identification need to be viewed with skepticism.

Step 2: Identification of What Is Desired

Once an assessment is made of what a particular corporate culture is, other questions can be asked: What is the corporate culture the organization would like to create? In our current organization, what are some of the corporate culture elements that need to be kept the same? What elements need to be changed, added to, or dropped? What does the organization need in order to survive in tomorrow's world? How do we keep ourselves from having a common shared purpose?

The exercise by Block on creating a vision of greatness can be usefully applied on the organizational level as well as on the individual and team levels. Take time to develop a vision of greatness for your organization. This becomes the what is desired.

Some of the areas to be considered are:

- Recruitment/selection
- Orientation
- Training
- Salary/benefits
- Career development and promotions
- Job design
- Employee assistance

Ask yourself what needs to be happening in these areas to bring about the vision of greatness you have for your organization.

Creating a vision of greatness is an exercise that can invite your organization to stretch. Do not hesitate to identify goals that you are not likely to reach immediately or may never reach. Such goals can still be useful in articulating a desired future.

Step 3: Planned Change for Corporate Culture

Once what is and what is desired have been determined, decision makers are in a position to make planned changes in the corporate culture so that the organization moves toward its vision of greatness. Note the concept of movement. The planned change process involves understanding the gaps between where an organization is and where it wants to be. With a clear understanding of those gaps, the organization can begin to find ways to increase its productivity and performance.

The process starts with a listing of statements such as here is where we are, here is what we desire, here are the steps we are taking in moving from what is to what is desired. However, for the process to be ultimately successful, the desired changes must be endorsed by top-level management. This is known as top-down modeling and is the most powerful way to tell the organization that the planned change is a serious effort.

Step 4: Monitoring the Planned Change Process

The planned change process must be monitored to see what is happening. One might ask whether the organization is moving in the desired direction. This movement may be quick, or it may be slow.

Part of the monitoring process is making mid-course corrections. As new influences come on the horizon, the institution can correct for them. Similarly, if targets are too easy, they can be stretched. In any case, each organization must decide for itself which methods of monitoring change are appropriate for the kind of change that is occurring.

The process of planned corporate culture is not new. However, what is new is the quest to identify and understand the organization's values and assumptions that have affected its productivity and performance. Once those values and assumptions have been identified, the organization can begin to build on its strengths and minimize its limitations.

Conclusion

Corporate culture is the earth in which the seeds of individual, team, and organizational performance and productivity are planted. If the earth is rich, then performance and productivity prosper. If not, the performance and productivity die off.

The purpose of this chapter has been to identify what corporate culture is and how it relates to performance and productivity at the individual, team, and organizational levels. In addition, the chapter has provided some techniques for assessing corporate culture and for redirecting that culture for high productivity and performance.

Farr (1985) has made an eloquent statement on organizational integrity that, for me, sums up the relationship of purpose, and hence commitment, to every organization:

> The essence of an organization is its purpose. Without the organizing force of purpose, there is no organization, there are merely people and things in random arrangement. The integrity of an organization, therefore, lies in the extent to which it operates "on purpose."

References

Adizes, I. *How to Solve the Mismanagement Crisis.* Homewood, IL: Dow Jones, Irwin, 1979.

Allaire, Y., and Firsirotu, M. Theories of organizational culture. *Organizational Studies* 5(3):1983, 1984.

Amsa, P. Organizational culture and work group behavior: an empirical study. *Journal of Management Studies* 23(3):347, May 1986.

Arnold, D., Capella, L., and Sumrall, D. Organizational culture and the marketing concept: diagnostic keys for hospitals. *Journal of Health Care Marketing* 7(1):18, Mar. 1987.

Atchison, T. Do you standout as a leader? *Healthcare Forum* 31(4):15, 1988.

Barney, J. Organizational culture: can it be a source of sustained competitive advantage? *Academy of Management Review* 11(3):656, July 1986.

Bates, P. The impact of organizational culture on approaches to organizational problem solving. *Organizational Studies* 5(1):43, 1984.

Block, P. *The Empowered Manager: Positive Political Skills at Work.* San Francisco: Jossey-Bass, 1987.

Clifton, Sr. R. Corporate culture and the healing mission. *Health Progress* 67(5):50, June 1986.

Desatnick, R. Management climate surveys: a way to uncover an organizational culture. *Personnel* 63(5):49, May 1986.

Farr, J. *Organizational Integrity.* Greensboro, NC: FARR Associates, 1985 (handout).

Flexner, W., and Gunkler, J. Confronting organizational change. *Healthcare Forum* 29(6):38, 1986.

Frankl, V. *Man's Search for Meaning.* New York City: Washington Square Press, 1963.

Gross, W., and Shichman, S. How to grow an organizational culture. *Personnel* 64(9):52, Sept. 1987.

Jones, J., and Bearley, W. *Organizational Change.* Bryn Mawr, PA: Organizational Design and Development, 1986.

Martin, J., and Siehl, C. Organizational culture and countercultures: an uneasy symbiosis. *Organizational Dynamics* 12(2):52, Autumn 1983.

Ouchi, W., and Wilkins, A. Organizational culture. *Annual Review of Sociology* 11:457, 1985.

Pareek, U. Dimensions of role efficiency. In: Jones, J., and Pfeiffer, W., editors. *1980 Handbook for Group Facilitators.* San Diego: University Associates, 1980.

Pennings, J., and Gresov, C. Technoeconomic and structural correlates of organizational culture: an integrative framework. *Organizational Studies* 7(4):317, 1986.

Reynierse, J., and Harker, J. Measuring and managing organizational culture. *Human Resource Planning* 9(1):1, 1986.

Schall, M. A communication-rules approach to organizational culture. *Administrative Science Quarterly* 28(4):557, Dec. 1983.

Schein, E. *Organizational Culture and Leadership.* San Francisco: Jossey-Bass, 1985.

Sherwood, J., and Glidewell, J. In: Jones, J., and Pfeiffer, W., editors. *The 1973 Annual Handbook for Group Facilitators.* San Diego: University Associates, 1973.

Ulschak, F. *Human Resource Development: The Theory and Practice of Needs Assessment.* Reston, VA: Reston Publishing, 1983.

Chapter 2

The Role of Management in Productivity and Performance Management

Vinod K. Sahney
Gail L. Warden

Introduction

The health care industry has undergone major changes during the past five years. The vocabulary of the industry is changing, with 1970s terms such as access to care, certificate of need, health systems agencies, rate review, and utilization review being replaced by new terms such as prospective pricing system (PPS), diagnosis-related group (DRG), preferred provider organization (PPO), managed care, health maintenance organization (HMO), price competition, low-cost delivery system, hospital marketing, case management, mergers, and vertical integration.

The health care industry is making a transition from a highly regulated, cost-based payment industry to a competitive price- and value-driven industry. This transition is not complete by any means, but the momentum for change is accelerating. Major payers such as Medicare and Medicaid have changed their payment systems from cost-based payment systems to prospective pricing systems. Managed care systems are negotiating with and selecting cost-effective providers. Business and industry are directly pressuring providers to be cost-competitive. These mounting pressures have forced providers to pay more attention to the cost of delivering health care services.

The authors wish to thank a number of colleagues who read the first draft of this manuscript and provided valuable comments. Special thanks are due R. Covert, A. Case, J. Dutkewych, B. Hoffmann, D. Klegon, M. Morris, D. Nerenz, I. Otis, P. Primeau, W. Schramm, and S. Velick.

No less intense are pressures in the area of quality of services. Customers are less willing to accept either long delays for appointments or long waits at physicians' offices. When health care organizations are faced with surplus capacity, customer service improvements become increasingly a part of institutional marketing strategies.

Given such an environment, what is the role of management in managing organizational performance? It is clear that the successful organizations during the next decade will be those that are able to master the art and science of productivity management. Here we define productivity broadly to include both the efficiency and the effectiveness with which health care services are delivered.

Productivity has been defined narrowly by economists as a ratio of output to input. Examples of labor productivity in a hospital under such a definition would include such measures as the number of laboratory tests performed per man-hour or the number of pounds of laundry processed per man-hour.

We use a broader definition: *productivity* is the quality, timeliness, and cost-effectiveness by which an organization achieves its mission. This definition implies that productivity improves as the quality of services is improved, even though the quantity of services remains the same. In addition, productivity improves when clinical effectiveness improves, such as when a physician is able to eliminate unnecessary testing or to treat patients in settings that are less resource-intensive with similar results.

How can we develop a productivity-driven organization? What is the role of management in creating such an environment? These are some of the issues we will discuss in this chapter. Before we address these issues, let us examine some typical situations faced by today's health care managers that illustrate the breadth of the productivity problem.

Productivity Management Situations

Consider the following situation faced by management across the country: XYZ Hospital has prided itself on being a full-service community hospital with 300 beds and an average occupancy of 70 percent. This hospital currently delivers 300 infants per year and has approximately 1,000 patient days in obstetrics. The census on the obstetrics unit varies from zero to eight on a given day; consequently, staffing needs vary greatly from day to day. The nursing staff feels that they do not have enough staff on many days, and nursing-staff productivity, when compared with national data for obstetrics units, is low. What can be done to enhance productivity? Let us examine some of the strategies available to management:

- *Strategy A: Manage Nursing Staffing.* The nursing director could ask the management engineering department to perform a nurse staffing study and suggest ways in which the nursing department could use a flexible staffing model to improve nursing productivity. A management engineer could also be asked to look at the work assignments of different employees in order to reduce the work load on nursing staff during peak periods.

- *Strategy B: Increase Marketing Effort.* The hospital has too few deliveries to maintain an efficient obstetrics unit. The hospital could plan and develop a major marketing campaign to increase the number of deliveries. The campaign could include improving the package of services made available to prospective mothers and increasing the number of community education programs.
- *Strategy C: Recruit Additional OB/GYN Medical Staff.* A third strategy open to the hospital is to recruit additional OB/GYN medical staff to the community that admits to this hospital. The hospital might attract other physicians by purchasing the practices of existing physicians that admit to a competitor hospital.
- *Strategy D: Contract with a Managed Care Program (HMO/PPO).* The hospital could contract with a managed care program for deliveries in a specified geographic region.
- *Strategy E: Close the Service.* The hospital has too few deliveries to maintain an efficient obstetrics unit. The hospital could close the obstetrics service.

Many other strategies are possible, but these five show a variety of ways that management might use to address the issue of productivity improvement. At one level (strategy A), the focus is on improving operations given the current volume of work. This is the focus of first-line supervisors and middle managers together with management engineers. At another level (strategies B through D), the focus is on strategies that will increase the volume of patients in the obstetrics unit, thus allowing the unit managers to improve the productivity of the staff by taking advantage of economies of scale as well as reduced fluctuations in volume. This is the focus of middle managers together with planning and marketing personnel. A successful campaign at this level has the potential for significantly improving labor productivity. Finally, strategy E addresses the product mix issue. If the hospital is unable to increase volume, it may eventually have to acknowledge that an efficient product line cannot be developed with the current volume. This is the focus of decision making at the top management level. The decisions made at this level will significantly affect organizational productivity.

Let us examine another situation: XYZ Hospital has experienced a loss of census of 11 percent during the past two years, from 78 percent in 1985 to 67 percent in 1987. Most of this decline is attributable to the reduction in length of hospital stay in the hospital across all payers. This hospital has 300 beds; it employed 1,250 employees in 1985 and now has 1,242 employees on the payroll. Hospital admissions have dropped from 14,600 in 1985 to

14,300 in 1987. Potential strategies to deal with this situation include the following:

- *Strategy X: Reduce Staff.* The hospital's chief financial officer could recommend that hospital management immediately order a layoff of 10 percent of employees across the board. This would allow the hospital to maintain a 4 percent profit on net revenue as the financial bottom line in 1988, the same as in 1985 before the downturn in census. He projects that unless layoffs take place, the hospital's financial bottom line may be a meager 1.5 percent of net revenue this year.
- *Strategy Y: Institute a Hiring Freeze, an Early Retirement Program, and Reduced Hours.* The chief human resources officer could recommend that the hospital not lay off employees. Her assessment of the situation is that employee morale would be negatively affected by a layoff. She suggests that the hospital immediately freeze hiring for all unfilled positions. An incentive package could be developed to encourage employees over 58 years of age to take voluntary early retirement. Another possible strategy is to allow employees to reduce their work hours in certain departments to 30 hours a week while maintaining full benefits.
- *Strategy Z: Set Employee Target Levels and Implement a Financial Incentive Plan.* The chief operating officer could recommend instituting a three-month period during which a target level would be set for 1988 and 1989 employee staffing levels with the assistance of department heads, supervisors, and management engineers. *Target level* is defined as the minimum number of employees needed to get the work done in order to meet the institution's financial bottom-line objectives. This staffing plan would then be presented to top-level management for approval. The plan would be used to set management objectives, and a financial incentive program would be tied to accomplishment of the objectives. In addition, all hospital employees would share in the financial rewards if the hospital met its targets.

Here again, management is faced with choices in addressing employee performance issues as well as the overall financial performance of the institution. A quick layoff would have an immediate impact on the financial bottom line. However, what would be the impact on morale, team-building efforts, and the hospital's future ability to attract technical staff? Could management ask employees to identify with the corporation and give 100 percent of effort in the future if job security were uncertain? What employee value system and culture is management trying to establish? Once again, we see that productivity management issues involve both the short- and long-range implications of management decisions.

We would like to emphasize that every decision of any significance made by hospital management ultimately affects organizational productivity and performance. These decisions involve such issues as product mix, capacity management, technology acquisition, product market share, and employee recruitment and training. Given the complexity of the productivity issue, it is important that management develop a comprehensive approach to managing productivity within the institution instead of riding currently popular bandwagons, such as idea systems, quality circles, productivity standards, or value improvement.

Hierarchy of Productivity Management

To improve productivity, management must focus its efforts and attention within the organization on several important levels. The three key levels are:

- Strategic focus
- Clinical effectiveness
- Operational efficiency

Strategic Focus

Strategic focus refers to the broadest set of goals, policies, and mission statements for an organization. Strategic focus is the responsibility of top-level management. Decisions at this level determine, to a great degree, the efficiency and effectiveness with which the health care organization deploys its aggregate resources to deliver and manage the care of the population it serves. At this level, decisions are made that define a framework for the organization's value system, its mission, and its culture. Customer service goals are set here. This is also where an organization makes critical decisions about product mix as well as new markets in which the organization will compete.

In developing a strategic focus, management needs to pay attention to the following key issues:

- Product mix
- Cost of individual product lines
- Management structure
- New product development
- Product quality

Defining product mix is crucial in productivity management. An organization must carefully study all of its product lines and those of its major competitors to decide which product lines it wishes to maintain, expand, or consolidate. Within each product line, the volume of services and the market share will determine whether the organization can effectively compete in the marketplace. During the cost-based reimbursement era, hospitals became accustomed to offering services even when the volume of services was too low to offer them economically. Under the prospective pricing system and in an increasingly competitive environment, institutions must study carefully the break-even volumes needed to offer a new service.

However, because hospitals are still a valuable community resource, product mix decisions should not be made in a vacuum. Community responsibility has to be considered. A rural hospital that is the only hospital in the service area may have to provide obstetrics services even if the volume does not justify it. Another example is care for AIDS patients, a financially unattractive product line but a needed service in many communities.

A second key issue for developing a strategic focus is the cost of various product lines. No health care organization can totally avoid the impact of inflation in the cost of supplies, utilities, liability insurance, and manpower, as well as the increasing cost of technology. Health care organizations need to carefully study the impact of increases in any of the above segments on their product lines as well as on those of their competitors. Health care organizations, especially tertiary care institutions, need to address all the ramifications of acquiring the increasingly costly health care technology that is continually introduced. For example, since new technology is introduced in community hospitals at a much slower pace than in tertiary care institutions, how can tertiary care hospitals compete with community hospitals for business in non–tertiary care admissions? There are limits to how much payers will pay to obtain the same product (say, herniotomy) at a teaching hospital versus a community hospital. Management needs to do a strategic cost analysis of the impact of the cost of inflation (Thompson, 1984) on the cost of producing health care. Strategies need to be developed that take into account the changes in cost structure (labor, supplies, and technology) in the health care industry. Management needs to analyze the cost structure of new technologies and programs and understand the economies of scale inherent in each of the new initiatives.

The third issue is that of management structure. Every organization needs to look at its structure periodically and ask itself: Are we organized in a way that is efficient and effective to accomplish the mission, goals, and objectives of the organization? Are decisions being made at the right level? Are people with product knowledge and familiarity making the key product decisions? Has the organization become too centralized, thus creating bottlenecks and second-guessing in decision making? Is the structure encouraging entrepreneurship and innovation while at the same time keeping controls in key delivery parameters of cost, quality, and service?

It is natural for top-level management to feel that the decisions must be made at the highest level. Even successful organizations drift toward centralization, sometimes by building a large corporate staff. Perhaps in response to this trend, two large corporations – IBM and General Electric – recently underwent major reorganizations to decentralize product decisions. In both cases, decision-making power was delegated to the product groups, and much of the corporate staff moved to lower levels of the hierarchy.

Today, health care managers need to pay particular attention to the organization's management structure because mergers, acquisitions, joint ventures, and diversification are becoming commonplace, and very little past experience exists either within the industry or on the part of the management. In such an environment, it is easy to build an overhead structure that is detrimental to performance improvement.

A productive organization is also one that looks toward introducing new and innovative products. The organization should develop a strategic focus that yields new products with an inherent, built-in advantage for the organization. As an example, if the institution currently serves a high percentage of elderly patients, a home health care company or a home equipment and supply company would be a natural product to develop. Similarly, an HMO or PPO might examine whether operating company-owned laboratory optical stores or pharmacies makes sense.

The general marketing strategy is to sell additional products to a current customer. This strategy has been well developed by makers of toys such as Legos, Atari video games, and Lionel electric trains. In each of these companies, the goal is to make the first sale, which is always the hardest sale. However, once people buy their first Lego set, for example, they are hooked. Soon they buy other related products. Health care organizations have the same opportunity to develop integrated product lines that allow the organization to take advantage of its base business and thus improve the efficiency and effectiveness with which new products are introduced in the marketplace.

Finally, top-level management needs to develop an obsession with product quality within the organization. Our broad definition of productivity, which implies that productivity improves as the quality of services is improved, encompasses the notion of providing value to the customer. Management needs to concentrate not only on developing the best diagnostic and treatment capabilities but also on providing the best service to patients.

Clinical Effectiveness

Most hospital resources consumed by patients are ordered by physicians (Young and Saltman, 1983). It is the physicians who decide how many diagnostic tests are needed to make or confirm diagnoses. Hence, successful productivity management programs must ensure that patients' cases are managed effectively by physicians and nurses while hospital management is worrying about how to produce services in the most cost-efficient manner. Hospital management does not need to use a great deal of mathematical wizardry to see where efforts can pay off: managers can reduce the cost of a diagnostic test by 10 percent from $40 to $36. But if a physician orders two tests instead of the one needed, the total cost per diagnosis goes up to $72 from $40, even with the increased production efficiency of 10 percent.

Clinical effectiveness is an area in which physicians and hospital management need to work together. Two major thrusts can be made to improve clinical effectiveness. The first involves information systems. Many tests are reordered because a patient's past test results are not available or were not sent by the referring physician or because the quality of the first one was poor. Many times, test results take too long to get back to units or get lost in the shuffle, and the physician ends up ordering a second battery.

A second thrust is the development of patient care protocols (Nackel and others, 1987). More groups of physicians need to discuss the optimum way to treat a patient. They should consider how long a patient needs to be in the hospital or when treatment can be shifted to a less resource-consuming environment, that is, a nursing home or even a patient's own home. Cataract surgery, which a few years ago almost routinely necessitated a three- or four-day hospital stay, now rarely requires a hospital stay. Similarly, patients undergoing antibiotic therapy and parenteral feedings are now routinely being treated at home by home infusion-therapy teams at less than 30 percent of the cost for hospital treatment.

To contribute to this second thrust, hospitals need to develop information systems that show resource utilization profiles by DRG by physician. These profiles should be studied to see why certain physicians use more resources to treat patients within the same DRG and the same severity of illness. Similarly, resource consumption in the clinical departments should be studied to see whether the material usage per ordered procedure is efficient. For example, how many X rays are retaken? In an intensive care unit, how many catheters are used to successfully place a Swan-Ganz catheter (Nackel and others, 1987)?

Operational Efficiency

Schermerhorn (1987) has challenged health care management to improve performance through high-performance managerial development. Performance can be defined as follows:

Performance = Employee ability × Systems support × Employee effort

For a health care system to achieve its maximum potential performance, top-level management must create an environment and a means by which each of the three key performance factors achieves its target. If the theoretical target for each factor is defined as 1.0 and an organization reaches 50 percent of its target in each of the three factors, the net performance level will only be 0.125 of its total accomplishment potential (0.5 × 0.5 × 0.5). Similarly, even if the organization achieves a goal of 1.0 in employee abilities and systems support, minimal employee efforts (say, 0.2 because of morale problems) will produce an institutional performance level of only 0.2 (1 × 1 × 0.2) of its maximum potential. Management must, therefore, pay attention to each of the three key factors simultaneously because the organization's performance will be limited by the weakest link in the chain.

Focusing on Employee Ability

Making the most of employee ability depends upon three factors: selection of employees, communication of expectations to employees, and development and training of employees. First and foremost is the selection of the employee. Most health care organizations pay insufficient attention to this factor, although other companies may give it thoughtful consideration. For example, Japanese auto companies building new plants in the United States (Mazda at Flat Rock, Michigan, and Nissan at Smyrna, Tennessee) put the plant workers through five to six levels of screening before accepting them as employees. Screening involves written tests and successive interviews by representatives of the human resources department, foremen, and management. The need to emphasize employee selection cannot be overemphasized.

The second factor that influences ability is setting performance expectations. Management must make a major effort to communicate clearly to employees what is expected of them in job performance. Here, management needs to set performance targets and review performance with employees on a regular basis.

The third factor is employee training and retraining. Management needs to develop employee training programs to provide opportunities for employees to improve their skills. These training programs must address every job. Examples of areas in which training programs can have a major impact include:

- Training programs for first-line supervisors in such topics as employee discipline, work scheduling, employee relations, and interviewing skills
- Training programs for receptionists in such areas as telephone answering skills, courtesy, and handling difficult patients, in addition to the job skills needed on an everyday basis
- Training and retraining of all employees as an ongoing effort, with regular evaluations of deficiencies and opportunities for improvement

Focusing on Support Systems

Another key performance factor for improving operational productivity is the development of support systems that encourage employees to achieve their full potential. Support systems encompass such areas as physical facilities, technology, management control systems, operations analysis support, and materials management.

An attractive and efficient work environment raises morale and increases the effectiveness of all employees. Management needs to pay attention to the work flow as well as to patient flow in a service area. Technical support from a physical facilities or operations analysis group may be needed to reorganize the area to ensure a smooth flow.

Another factor that should be considered is technology, which includes administrative systems and equipment. Among these systems are such institutionwide systems as patient registration, medical record index, patient appointment, and billing, just to name a few. The ease of using these systems will affect the productivity of every area within the organization.

Management control systems that also need to be examined include budgeting systems, cost-accounting systems, productivity monitoring systems, employee evaluation systems, and position control systems. It is important that the management control systems be interlinked and consistent with each other; no system should work in a vacuum. For example, a position control system needs to be tied to the annual budgeting cycle. It needs to address not only the number of positions but also the desired level of skills for each position. It is not unusual for "skill inflation" to take place over a period of time. Each opening must be looked upon as an opportunity to evaluate the skill levels needed for the job. One continually needs to ask, could this be done effectively by a person with less education and experience? Do we really need a registered nurse for this position, or could a medical assistant successfully perform this job? Similarly, how are new positions approved? What is the linkage of the approval process to the budgeting system and the productivity monitoring system?

A credible system for monitoring labor productivity must be installed (Serway and others, 1987; Kelliher, 1985). The focus, however, should not be on absolute standards. In a health care delivery system, the product is highly variable and labor-intensive, making the establishment of absolute standards difficult. Hence, it is better to focus on a process of continual improvement rather than to argue for ultimate standards. Management needs to set up an environment in which the management engineering effort focuses on providing consultative assistance to the department managers on how to improve productivity rather than on evaluation and punishment. Simultaneously, individual department-based tools for measuring the quality of services should be developed. Quality of services should be defined both to patients and to other users of services, including physicians and other departments.

Operations analysis support can include the management of patient flow and demand in health care organizations (Eastaugh, 1985). In health care, as in many service industries, demand for services varies by the time of day and the day of the week. In general, health care managers have not paid sufficient attention to alternative strategies for managing the variability in demand, but instead have relied on either peak-level staffing or working for stretches of time understaffed (Griffith and others, 1976).

Sahney (1982) discussed a series of strategies that address the variability in demand, including strategies to influence the demand generation process and to adjust the service capacity on the basis of work load needs. Management's first priority should be to influence the demand generation process whenever possible. The foremost strategy here is to use a reservation system or its variations to distribute the demand more evenly. A clinic appointment system and operating room case scheduling are two examples of this strategy. Department-level managers need to study demand patterns by time of day and day of the week and to use this information to alter schedules whenever possible. A significant demand for services in health care organizations is created by elective admissions. It is, therefore, important that management pay attention to managing the fluctuations in patient census. Sahney (1974) and Hancock and others (1978) described elective admission scheduling procedures to manage patient census. These systems not only even out the patient census but also help to reduce cancellations of both elective admissions and surgeries.

Other strategies to manage demand include matching complementary demand (matching demand in two different areas where the demand peaks at different times in each area; for example, outpatient pharmacy demand may peak between 10:00 a.m. and 2:00 p.m., whereas inpatient pharmacy demand peaks between 7:00 and 10:00 a.m.). Management can minimize the variability in demand by looking for methods to change patient behavior, such as publishing in patient newsletters the best times to call for appointments or urgent visits or asking patients to call in the morning and ask the nurse what is the best time for walk-in patients to see a physician.

If demand cannot be evenly distributed, strategies to alter service capacity need to be put in place. When demand peaks are known and predictable, the use of part-time employees is effective. If demand peaks are unpredictable, one can use overtime and work-priority setting to manage demand. Cross-training can be used to handle peak levels for both predictable and unpredictable situations. For slow periods of demand, incentive time-off strategies can bring the service capacity down to match the demand. (For example, a hospital can encourage staff to take vacation time during low census by counting only a half-day for each full day taken as vacation.) By using a combination of strategies to manage demand as well as service capacity, a health care manager can keep quality of service up while maintaining a high level of productivity among staff (Sahney, 1982).

Finally, support systems need to address the nonmanpower issues that affect operational efficiency. In health care organizations, the cost of materials and supplies accounts for 20 to 30 percent of costs. A strong materials management and supply control system needs to be designed together with an effective purchasing system. The use of group purchasing systems is well documented in the industry and is practiced widely. Little attention, however, has been given to inventory management at the user level. Stockpiling in supply closets often results in turning over inventory less than once per year.

Focusing on Employee Effort

The overall level of employee effort, the third key performance factor, depends a great deal on the individual employee's motivation to give extra effort on the job. An important strategy in improving employee morale and encouraging extra effort is to build on the concept of the team. The less the distinction between management and workers, the more the opportunity to develop the team concept. Japanese manufacturers with plants in the United States have effectively demonstrated this concept (New York Stock Exchange Office of Economic Research, 1982). In U.S. auto plants, separate dining rooms for management-level employees are common, but Japanese plants in the United States have a single dining facility for management and workers. In Japanese plants in the United States, all employees wear the same uniform as the shop workers. The uniform minimizes the class distinction between members of the same team. Another strategy for building the team concept is to have sports teams or community projects sponsored by the organization. Through these efforts all employees can get behind their organization and develop a sense of pride and ownership not unlike the pride a sports team generates within a university or a city. A multitude of potential intervention strategies can be implemented on the basis of organizational needs to promote team achievement effectively.

A second strategy for increasing employee motivation is to tie rewards to performance whenever possible. At the institutionwide level, a profit-sharing program can be instituted to distribute a pool of dollars on the basis of institutional performance. At the departmental level, profit-sharing programs can be designed in a manner that rewards members of individual departments for reaching departmental as well as institutional goals. One such program is "Improshare," which was developed by Mitchell Fein (1983) and is currently being used in more than 200 manufacturing corporations. More recently, this concept has been applied to health care. The first application of "Improshare" in the health care field was at John F. Kennedy Hospital in New Jersey (Fein, 1985). The key design concepts can be summarized as follows:

- Every member of the organization is important and needed.
- Employees can contribute to improvement.
- Productivity increases with recognition and sharing.
- The reasons for rewards should be fair and understandable to all.
- Employees and the organization share equally in all productivity gains.
- Productivity gains are measured at the organizational level.
- Individual departments qualify to share in the productivity gains at the organizational level by meeting or beating departmental targets.

Besides financial rewards, recognition and praise can be great motivators. Employee of the month programs and best departmental performance awards are tools that can be effectively used to increase employee motivation. An example of this is demonstrated by a Sunnyvale, California, hightech corporation. Near the entrance to the company headquarters is a reserved parking place with a sign that says Employee of the Month. The name of the employee of the month is etched on the sign, and for one month, that is the assigned spot for the selected employee. At almost no cost to the organization, public recognition is being given to the best employees. Another example of employee recognition is the annual employee recognition dinner at Henry Ford Hospital in Detroit. Employees and their families are invited to a semiformal dinner dance when they reach 15, 20, 25, 30, 35, 40, 45, or 50 years of service with the organization. At the Nissan plant in Smyrna, Tennessee, employees in the best department (determined by records of the quality of production for a year) are invited along with their families to a black-tie dinner. This dinner is personally served by members of top-level management.

Employee motivation can also be increased by facilitating upward job mobility within the organization. At Henry Ford Hospital, all jobs must be posted within the corporation for a fixed period before outside recruiting is started. In addition, this hospital offers extensive educational programs through which employees can improve their work skills and compete effectively for job promotions. Tuition assistance and encouragement to improve one's educational background are other ways to help employees to move up to more challenging jobs.

Strategies such as building the concept of the team, linking rewards to performance, and giving recognition and praise are not sufficient by themselves to create a motivated team. However, by conveying a sense that the organization sincerely cares about its employees, these strategies reinforce each other, thus creating a positive environment in which the members of the organization feel willing to give an extra effort on behalf of the organization.

A third strategy for improving employee motivation is to ensure two-way communication among all levels of employees. Such communication must take place between employees and supervisors on a daily and weekly basis. Similarly, newsletters for employees and their families that discuss major initiatives taken by the organization and its successes and anticipated difficulties are another way to keep members of the organization informed. In addition, management should set aside time for small-group, face-to-face meetings with all employees. These meetings should provide opportunities for employees to share their thoughts with the organization's leadership.

The Role of the Chief Executive Officer

What is the role of the chief executive officer (CEO) in productivity management? Clearly, the CEO's role is not at the operational level. It is not the

CEO's job to define productivity for each department or, for'that matter, to measure the output of individual departments. Neither is it the CEO's job to worry about patient flow or efficient scheduling methods. This is best left to individual department heads and management engineers. Similarly, it is not the CEO's job to design patient-care protocols. These are best left to the medical staff and to utilization review and quality assurance departments.

The CEO's job is to provide leadership in productivity improvement. It is his or her job to provide an environment in which managers and physicians are motivated to constantly improve the current system. It is the CEO's job to periodically examine the product mix and to ask strategic questions about what business the organization is in and, more important, what business it should be in. Major product mix or market-entry decisions will have a significant effect on productivity, and this is where the chief executive officer can have a major impact. Decisions at this level need vision and foresight, and analysis can only be partially helpful.

Another area in which the CEO can have a major impact on productivity is in examining the organization's structure as well as the ability of its management team. Does the current structure enable the organization to implement productivity improvements? Does the structure motivate innovation and entrepreneurship? Do the senior managers work as a team, or are individuals more concerned about who gets the credit? Are critical decisions discussed with input from key areas, and are decisions to move forward made without constant second-guessing? The development of a senior management policy group is a key responsibility of the CEO.

Finally, it is the CEO who, by setting an appropriate example and providing leadership, will develop a culture and value system within the organization. Once members of the organization understand that increased productivity is the long-term solution to profitability, the barriers to productivity improvement can be addressed one by one.

Conclusion

Productivity and performance management is a prime imperative for the 1990s. In this chapter we have discussed a number of strategies for improving productivity and institutional performance. Management needs to address three key levels simultaneously in order to improve productivity on a continual basis. These levels are strategic focus, clinical effectiveness, and operational efficiency. The chief executive officer needs to set the tone and framework in which productivity improvement plays a key role within the organization.

We end this chapter by listing the basic strategies for improving productivity:

- Define the product mix.
- Understand economies of scale.
- Determine a framework for delivering high-quality services.
- Manage demand variability.
- Manage service capacity.
- Manage the acquisition of technology.
- Understand the impact of cost inflation.
- Manage employee development.
- Manage employee involvement.
- Measure and monitor productivity improvement.
- Pay attention to consumer needs.
- Reevaluate organizational structure.
- Create an environment for innovation.
- Develop a process for employee recognition and rewards.
- Make productivity and quality a religion, an integral part of management and the organizational decision-making process.

References

Eastaugh, S. R. Improving hospital productivity under PPS: managing cost reductions. *Hospital and Health Services Administration* 30(4):97–111, July–Aug. 1985.

Fein, M. Improved productivity through worker involvement. *Industrial Management* 25(3):1–12, May–June 1983.

Fein, M. Raising productivity of hospitals by sharing productivity gains. Unpublished paper, Mitchell Fein, Inc., Hillsdale, NJ, 1985.

Griffith, J. R., Hancock, W. M., and Munson, F. C. *Cost Controls in Hospitals.* Ann Arbor, MI: Hospital Administration Press, 1976, pp. 330–31.

Hancock, W. M., Warner, D. M., Heda, S., and Fuho, P. Admission scheduling and control systems. In: Griffiths, J. R., Hancock, W. M., and Munson, F. C., editors. *Cost Control in Hospitals.* Ann Arbor, MI: Health Administration Press, 1978, pp. 150–85.

Kelliher, M. E. Managing productivity, performance and the cost of services. *Healthcare Financial Management* 39(9):23–28, Sept. 1985.

Nackel, J. G., Kis, G. M., and Fernaroli, P. J. *Cost Management for Hospitals.* Rockville, MD: Aspen Publications, 1987, p. 245.

New York Stock Exchange Office of Economic Research. *People and Productivity: A Challenge to Corporate America.* New York City: New York Stock Exchange Office of Economic Research, 1982.

Sahney, V. K. Using evolutionary information for effective admission scheduling. *Proceedings: Conference on Patient Scheduling.* Washington, DC: American Hospital Association, Nov. 18–19, 1974, pp. 19–41.

Sahney, V. K. Managing variability in demand: a strategy for productivity improvement in health care services. *HCM (Health Care Management) Review* 7(2):37–41, Spring 1982.

Schermerhorn, J. R. Improving health care productivity through high performance managerial development. *HCM (Health Care Management) Review* 12(4):49–56, Fall 1987.

Serway, G. D., Strum, D. W., and Haug, W. F. Alternative indicators for measuring hospital productivity. *Hospital and Health Services Administration* 32(3):379–98, Aug. 1987.

Thompson, A. A. Strategies for staying cost competitive. *Harvard Business Review* 62(1):110–17, Jan.–Feb. 1984.

Young, D. W., and Saltman, R. B. Preventive medicine for hospital costs. *Harvard Business Review* 61(1):126–33, Jan.–Feb. 1983.

Chapter 3

Management Systems: A Key Part of the Productivity Strategy

Raymond A. Buttaro
Alan J. Goldberg

Introduction

Productivity depends on many factors that are typically analyzed separately, although they are interrelated. Because productivity depends on many variables, productivity improvements often are not attained or are only partially implemented. Similarly, the benefits of major capital expenditures for modernizing facilities, implementing computerization, or acquiring new equipment or technology often are not as great as anticipated. Worse yet, improvements in one area may be realized at the expense of quality, service levels, or increased work load in another area. In many cases, work load and staffing needs are actually increased drastically as a result of supposed productivity improvement programs. Such issues affect the organization's efficiency at both the corporate level (or macrolevel) and the departmental level (or microlevel). Unless the productivity strategy addresses the full spectrum of the institution's needs (including labor, materials, and quality issues) on both levels, lasting improvements cannot be realized.

An organization's physical environment is just one factor limiting productivity. An organization's wage and salary program, policies and procedures, organizational structure, and information management system typically have a greater impact on productivity than does the physical plant. For maximum and lasting productivity improvements, every productivity improvement strategy must encompass the total organization. Such an organizationwide approach should include the following steps:

- Establishing a real commitment to productivity by educating managers

- Conducting an operational audit and a management systems review
- Conducting a facilities review
- Monitoring performance
- Linking productivity with compensation

When examined in the context of productivity, many management systems and organizational structures in common use prove ineffective. When systems in which productivity is a key element are implemented, such management systems can play a major role in an organization's productivity strategy.

Education and Commitment

A health care organization must be committed to its strategy for improving productivity if it is to derive any lasting benefit from productivity improvements. The education and commitment phase of a productivity strategy should encompass all facets of the productivity mix, including labor, supplies, facilities, service levels, and quality. Improvements in productivity should start with developing a common data base to ensure consistency and allow for monitoring progress. Elements of this common data base should include the following:

- *Definitions:* Terms and concepts should be accurately defined for all users of the data base. Sources of data and reporting responsibilities also must be established. The number of worked hours may have a different meaning depending on the user's reference point. Is time spent off-site at a conference considered part of the worked hour total? Is the information source departmental records or payroll records? When and to whom are the data to be reported?
- *Goals:* The organization's goals and objectives related to productivity should be clearly identified. This enables line managers, for example, to develop appropriate productivity strategies. In addition, establishing and communicating corporate productivity goals emphasize the significance of the issue for employees on all levels.
- *Responsibilities:* Responsibility for specific productivity activities should be assigned to staff members. Specified times should be established for both ongoing (that is, preparation of periodic productivity reports) and single-occurrence activities.
- *Uses of the Information:* As part of the initial phase of the productivity effort, employees should gain an understanding of how productivity data will be used. Because productivity data are often integrated with other departmental information such as cost-accounting, pricing, and budgeting data and data from quality-monitoring activities, productivity data must be accurate. Linking the manager's salary

reviews with productivity performance is one strategy for maximizing productivity.

Once these initial steps are under way, the most beneficial next phase is the education of management-level personnel. Depending on the organization's goals, the length of this education phase can vary from 2 to 16 hours of classroom presentation. During this time, specific productivity concepts should be reviewed and current productivity issues should be discussed. In addition, educational sessions are an ideal time to restate the organization's productivity goals and progress to date.

Many educational programs are available for management training in productivity. The key is selecting one that is in sync with the needs of the organization and the capabilities of line managers and is appropriate for the anticipated uses of the productivity information. For example, an educational program appropriate for a detailed standards-setting, productivity-monitoring, and cost-accounting effort would be inappropriate for a system meant to monitor quick trends.

In any event, executive management must participate in the educational effort. This participation reinforces the organization's commitment to the program and establishes a corporate mind-set as a model for line managers to follow. In many instances, nonmanagement employees participate in the program by acting as case leaders or presenters, by responding to managers' questions, or both.

The topics to be discussed in any presentation should include:

- The organization's goals
- The history of productivity (national, industrywide, and organizational)
- The importance of productivity
- Techniques for improving productivity
- Expectations of management
- Techniques for setting standards
- Procedures used in the reporting system
- Quality issues
- Supply usage

Many health care organizations have found that the implementation of a formal employee suggestion program serves as an excellent start for the education effort. The suggestion program gets employees thinking about methods to improve operations and encourages change by establishing a reward system. Elements of a good suggestion program include the following:

- *A Specified Time Period:* The program should be planned for a short, clearly identified time period (that is, two to six weeks). Appropriate in-house and external publicity must be timed to coincide with the program dates.

- *Rewards for All Who Submit Suggestions:* A reward system encourages participation.
- *The Capacity to Investigate and Analyze the Benefits of Each Suggestion:* The group assigned the task of evaluating the suggestions offered by employees should include management analysts if possible. The evaluation criteria should be communicated to all participants, thus eliminating postprogram concerns regarding favoritism.
- *A Willingness to Implement Appropriate Suggestions:* Failure to implement valid suggestions results in decreased participation in and acceptance of future productivity programs.

With these initial phases completed, the organization will have established and communicated its goals for productivity, established a common data base, and educated managers on the issues related to productivity. As a result, hospital managers should be working in harmony with the corporate goals and should be receptive to implementing changes. The next phase is to identify factors that limit productivity gains, decrease efficiency, or both.

Operational Audit

Many factors affect productivity, including facilities, layout, support systems, and job descriptions. When these factors are in tune with management's productivity goals, implementing changes and improving productivity are relatively easy. When they are at odds with the goals, however, improvements in productivity are unlikely to occur unless levels of service or quality are decreased.

How can management quickly and cost-effectively assess the status of the organization's systems and current productivity performance? Applied Management Systems (AMS) has found that the operational audit is a cost-effective process for establishing baseline data and assessing the efficiency and effectiveness of current operating systems. Just as financial records must be periodically audited to ensure their accuracy and adherence to sound accounting principles, so too must the operating and support systems be periodically reviewed to ensure that they are in accordance with sound productivity principles.

The audit is a brief but intensive review of all operations and productivity levels. In this AMS approach, the audit team (which consists of three to five functional/area specialists versed in health care operations) spends approximately one week on-site. During this time the team reviews operational specifics with department managers, develops a sensitivity to organizational specifics, and meets with appropriate line and executive management staff. The end result is a general assessment of each department's operational status and an audit of the organization's operations, including staffing, equipment and facility limitations, comparative data, recommended productivity standards, and adequacy of support systems.

The audit enables management to establish priorities and finalize productivity strategies. Three areas that hinder productivity goals are generally identified:

- Human resources
- Organizational structure
- Facilities

Typically, the status of at least one of these areas impedes efficiency and limits productivity.

Human Resources

Human resources policy and practice have a significant impact on operations. The term *human resources* as used here includes:

- Wage and salary programs
- Staffing
- Scheduling

The wage and salary program of a health care organization is an integral part of the productivity mix. The key points that should be noted are the following:

- Position descriptions should not limit the flexibility and productivity goals of management.
- The position description should be a description of the actual job, not a typical assignment schedule.
- The position grade should be based on job factor evaluation (that is, educational experience, manual skills, physical environment, manual effort, supervisory responsibility, and so forth).
- Salary surveys should be undertaken to ensure that competitive wages are being offered.
- Periodic staff salary reviews must include productivity performance as one of the evaluation criteria.
- The wage and salary program should be part of the organization's strategy for productivity gains.

Policies guiding staffing and scheduling should be part of the total productivity strategy. Often, policy precludes staffing for high levels of productivity. For example, policies may be based on situations that no longer exist.

During a recent operational audit at a hospital, for example, a review of the staff scheduling policy was found to be counterproductive to efficiency.

The hospital had established a schedule that did not allow the scheduling of vacations during the Christmas–New Year's period (approximately December 15 through January 1). The policy had been established during the late 1960s in response to census and acuity levels, physician practice patterns, and nursing availability. It was still in effect in the middle 1980s even though the situation had changed significantly. At the time of the audit, the census level exhibited a significant decrease over the holidays. After January 1, when the census level returned to normal, staff requested time off. Thus, the hospital's scheduling policy conflicted with the working situation. A simple change in vacation policy resulted in increased productivity, improved morale, lower staff turnover, reduced costs, and improved patient care.

Organizational Structure

The organizational structure of a health care organization has a significant effect on productivity. An effectively structured organization faces minimal communication problems, work duplication, and conflicts. Implementing needed changes in both the formal and informal organizational structure is simple in such organizations.

Many health care organizations have implemented materials management concepts—centralized purchasing, storage, and distribution. Upon close scrutiny, however, it is evident that many departments in these organizations are not a part of the centralized system. In reality, these departments have a decentralized system of materials management, which decreases productivity even though the formal organization exhibits true materials management.

In many other instances, an organization's structure does not support productivity. These include the following:

- *Transportation:* Transportation systems are often decentralized, with individual departments meeting their own patient transport needs. This results in unnecessary trips and often employs scarce staff (registered nurses, therapists, and technicians) for routine transport. When there is a centralized service in place, appropriate guidelines must be established to ensure cost-effective service. All too often there is little scheduling of demand attempted, which results in poor quality of service and peak demands that are difficult to meet.
- *Patient Scheduling:* The scheduling of services in most ancillary departments is done for the convenience of the department or the physicians rather than in response to patients' needs or patient volume. Examination scheduling is a logical, inexpensive way to maximize staff and facility resources while meeting the demand for services.
- *Information Systems:* At one time, fears were commonplace that computerization would eliminate jobs. All too often, because of poor planning or incomplete implementation, the advent of a computer has

actually increased work load, usually because management systems were not changed to conform to the computer's capabilities. Record duplication, manual data inputs and transfers, and poor placement of workstations are some of the causes of increased work load.

Although centralization of functions or support services often results in improved operational efficiency, centralization should not be viewed as a panacea for inefficiency. Other factors must be assessed to design the most cost-effective solution to the specific need. Such factors include:

- Minimum staffing needs that result in low productivity (work that could be transferred to a central service may not necessarily improve productivity)
- Service needs that may dictate decentralized support (secretarial, transport, and so forth) to meet the unique demands placed on a department

The key is the end result. If throughout the institution maximum efficiency is being realized with a smoothly functioning decentralized system, the benefits of centralization may be minimal.

Facilities

Productivity problems associated with the physical facilities of departments in health care organizations are the most difficult to correct, and they represent a costly impediment to productivity goals. The areas to be looked at in assessing physical facilities include:

- The location of the department
- The condition of the facilities
- The department's proximity to related departments or areas
- The appropriateness of the equipment within the department
- The size of the area
- The layout of the area
- Off-site departmental space
- Workflow patterns

The following space analysis principles can be applied:

- *Space is a limited resource for health care organizations, especially given the regulatory environment and the high cost of construction.* Although the costs associated with space (interest and depreciation) account for approximately 6 to 8 percent of health care costs, the health care organization must carefully manage this limited resource. Under the current regulatory mandates (certificate of need, reimbursement, zoning, and so forth), it is often difficult to obtain additional space. Therefore, the space needed for each department and its activity should be as carefully scrutinized as the staffing levels needed. Often, such an analysis can reveal ways to reallocate existing space to meet current needs without expansion. Also, once facilities are built, they must be maintained, thus adding to operating costs.

- *Bottlenecks may exist that have an impact on overall operations.* One important aspect of analyzing facilities is to determine whether any bottlenecks are caused by the current facilities. For example, does the facility have the right number of operating rooms? If not, perhaps the queue for surgery has a negative effect on ancillary departments, the admitting department, and the emergency room.

- *The layout and relationships among departments greatly affect overall productivity.* An analysis of the physical flow of personnel, patients, materials, and information often can reveal opportunities for increased efficiencies. For example, the size or layout of a nursing station may require high staffing levels because of the length of the floor or the visual inaccessibility of certain areas. Areas for two closely related activities (the emergency room and the radiology department) may be separated by a distance that results in excessive transporting of patients back and forth.

- *In measuring departmental efficiency, the space required to perform the activity should be included.* Most department heads focus only on their budgeted direct costs in examining their overall productivity. However, each department is directly responsible for the space it uses as well. Because the amount of space used is within the control of the department head, the department head should make trade-offs among space, labor, and material to ensure optimal utilization of all resources. If Department A performs the same activities as Department B but in twice as much space, then, all other things being equal, Department A is less productive. It uses more resources to produce the same level of output.

The first step in analyzing the productivity factor of physical facilities is to determine whether the facilities are adequate to meet the needs of the personnel and patients who use them. The second step is to determine whether the facilities are well utilized. These two factors must be analyzed in a unified approach. Obviously, we could easily satisfy ourselves on one point if we totally abandoned the other. For example, if there were only one operating room when five were needed, excellent utilization would be ensured; however, the users' needs (those of the physicians and patients) would probably not be met in a timely fashion. Thus, the goal is to arrange the best compromise possible between utilization and needs.

Several operations research techniques have been applied in the health care setting to resolve facility analysis issues. The techniques range from the sophisticated to the simple. Included among these are:

- Simulation programs that forecast the impact of various changes
- Queuing theory techniques that balance customer waiting times
- Linear programming to optimize allocation of resources
- Workflow analysis

Although these sophisticated approaches may require special knowledge, computer programs, or both, it is often wise to use them to attain maximum benefit.

Many simple approaches are often applicable as well. Even in the application of simple techniques, it is important to include three variables in the analysis:

- *Volume:* How many units of service must be handled by the facility?
- *Time Requirements:* How much facility time will be needed for each unit of service?
- *Facility Capacity:* How much time is made available by each facility unit?

For example, to determine the required number of operating rooms, it is necessary to know:

- How many procedures are performed by procedure type
- How long each procedure type takes
- How much time is available for each available room

It is important that the layout does not serve to hinder the operations being performed. Sometimes a change in layout can free up a bottleneck or obviate the need for additional space.

These approaches to facility review can be best illustrated with case examples. The first case deals with the construction of new facilities, the second with the redesign of existing facilities, and the third with minor modifications of existing facilities.

Case 1: New Facility Construction

The current hospital facility is 20 to 60 years old, is not in compliance with codes, and is in need of major repair or replacement. The hospital has also been experiencing serious overcrowding resulting from increases in service demands.

As part of the master plan, the architects developed design alternatives. Initially, five basic designs were under consideration; two were eliminated by the administrative staff. One design that was rejected involved the refurbishing of the present facility and would not be in total compliance with the current life-safety guidelines; the other design was deemed to be too costly. The three remaining plans were turned over to the management systems professionals for review and comment. However, the systems staff requested that all five plans be subjected to their screening process to ensure optimal layout selection.

A six-faceted screening process was developed to review the plans. The factors considered were:

- Initial cost
- Compliance with the various regulations and guidelines
- Staffing costs
- Layouts of the departments
- Operating costs
- Financial analysis (return on investment, payback, and so forth)

The interaction between hospital functional areas was analyzed. Such factors as trip frequency and skill involvement were documented under the present layout. Each alternative was then compared with the revised travel distance to optimize the layout. Such factors as number and location of elevators and storage areas and departmental location were considered in this review.

The staffing costs were documented for factors such as:

- The nursing requirements under each layout
- The housekeeping requirements under each layout
- The time requirement for performing portable radiology procedures under each layout
- The maintenance requirements of each layout
- The dietary, labor, and equipment requirements under each layout
- The central supply costs under each layout
- The accessibility for laboratory technicians under each layout
- The messenger/transporter needs under each layout
- The materials distribution (labor and equipment needs) under each layout

To complete the life-cycle analysis, such ongoing operational costs as projected inventory levels, equipment needs, and energy consumption were considered. The final result was that the most expensive building plan with the highest construction costs was the most cost-effective over the projected life of the facility.

In this process, the building committee of the hospital board discussed the concepts and operational systems changes without consideration for their impact on work load. An example of this was their decision to implement a case cart resupply system in the surgical suite. To the architect, case carts meant an alcove for cart storage within the surgical suite, not a total revamping of the activities and responsibilities of the Central Supply Department. However, under the organizational structure in place, central supply duties were the responsibility of the operating room. As part of their duties, the operating room staff cleaned and prepared the instruments after a case and selected the instruments and supplies in preparation for the next day's cases. Once the equipment needs, work load and staffing reassignments, space reallocations, revised charging and ordering systems, and transfer of responsibilities were documented, the new system was implemented with a minimum of confusion and delay.

Case 2: Redesign of Existing Facility

With the opening of its new 15-bed emergency facility, a hospital experienced major unanticipated problems with patient delays, paperwork flow, billing, staffing, and supply usage. To address these problems, a complete systems study was undertaken to assist the hospital in treating its annual 45,000-patient caseload.

A review of the delay sites revealed that the new, long-awaited physical plant was not conducive to smooth, effective patient flow. In addition, the emergency department design did not allow for the proper mix of rooms, for the proper monitoring of supply storage areas, or for functional paperwork systems.

Major study recommendations included renovation to allow for improved paper and patient flow, reassignment of rooms, changes in the patient charging system, and a complete redesign of the emergency medical record. In addition, with the data available, a flexible staff scheduling system was designed to coincide with patient loads. Finally, monitoring systems were implemented to track both room and staff utilization on an ongoing basis. After the changes were implemented, average patient time through the emergency room decreased from 75 minutes to 30 minutes, staffing decreased by 4.6 full-time equivalents, charge capture accuracy increased by approximately 60 percent, and paperwork was significantly reduced (through the consolidation of forms, the modification of flow, and the elimination of the duplicative system). The flow before analysis was:

1. Patient arrival logged by receptionist
2. Assessment sheet completed by assessment nurse
3. Assessment sheet brought to transient admitting
4. Emergency medical record completed by transient admitting
5. Assessment sheet and record brought to nursing station
6. Assessment sheet and record brought to examination/treatment room
7. As needed, requisitions completed by transient admitting and brought to the nursing station

The flow after analysis was:

1. Patient to assessment
2. Assessment data entered on chart by nurse

3. Chart handed to admitting clerical (if routine patient) and patient directed to a transient admitting station
4. Admission completed by typist
5. Patient waits for treatment

As a result of these changes, the hospital was able to maximize the usefulness of a poorly designed facility without a major capital expenditure. Ideally, these issues would have been addressed in the original design; however, all too often, new facilities result in increased work load. With sound workflow analysis, systems can be adapted to the facility design.

Case 3: Radiology Suite in Older Facility

The radiology suite in an older facility was experiencing low productivity resulting from lengthy examination processing times, delays, and poor workflows. Because there was little funding available for major renovation or construction and because the work load did not warrant any staff increases, it became necessary for the department to look for better methods within current constraints. Three problems found in the layout of the department are described below.

- The department was arranged backwards. Patients entered from the rear of the department and traveled to the front of the department, where the reception and waiting room was located. Outpatients walked past inpatients who were waiting in the radiology corridor.
- There were no patient direction signs when one entered the department from the main corridor. There was no sign to indicate that the patient had entered the Radiology Department.
- Patients walking into the Radiology Department often stopped at the technologist station/darkroom to ask for directions. The technologist verified the patient's name on the radiology schedule and directed the patient to the reception desk. The person at the reception desk greeted the patient and notified the technologist that the patient had arrived, even though the technologist already had seen the patient.

The evaluation of patient flow and department layout resulted in the following recommendations:

- Adequate patient direction signs should be installed to identify the Radiology Department and direct patients to the reception desk.
- Signs should also be posted to indicate the individual sections within the Radiology Department. The patient reception area should have a sign that is visible to patients walking down the radiology corridor.
- The patient reception area should be relocated to the entrance to the Radiology Department.

The hospital is now considering a modest renovation program to re-design the department to allow for effective patient, paper, and staff flows. In addition, extensive revisions to the transportation, filing, transcription, and examination scheduling systems have indicated sufficient cost savings to justify these renovations.

Conclusion Based on Case Studies

In all of the preceding cases, the problems could have been avoided if perfect planning had occurred. In the real world, perfection seldom occurs, and this is where facility and systems analysis enters. The goal is to maximize the effectiveness and efficiency of the facility within the health care organization's physical and financial limitations.

Performance

Performance monitoring is the keystone of any productivity improvement effort. Without some sort of performance reporting system, improvement is difficult, if not impossible. With performance monitoring, improvement is at least feasible, although not guaranteed. The diligence with which health care managers monitor productivity is directly related to the productivity levels attained by the staff. The monitoring system is the final link in the management system strategy.

There are many types and uses of performance monitoring systems. A sampling of types of systems includes:

- Budgets, fixed or variable
- MONITREND (the Hospital Administrative Services/MONITREND Reporting Service)
- Standards-based systems
- Comparison-based systems
- Position control
- Payroll reports

It is important to use the system or systems already available in the organization. Health care managers must ensure that the reports are timely, accurate, auditable, understandable, and usable.

Many health care organizations make the mistake of not tracking performance because there is no system available to do so or because the system available is not state-of-the-art. This situation represents as serious a mistake as not monitoring at all, and it is tantamount to not managing performance.

The system used does not have to be complicated or all-embracing, but it must be used! An example of a simple system is a trend-based system.

In such a system, baseline data are established and performance is tracked against this baseline. Examples of informative ratios appropriate for trending are:

- Days in accounts receivable
- Care hours per patient day (CHPPD)
- Radiology examinations per technician worked hour
- Laboratory CAP (College of American Pathologists) units per paid hour

Sample results of a CHPPD trend are as follows:

Month:	Oct.	Nov.	Dec.	Jan.	Feb.	Mar.	Apr.	May	June	July	Aug.	Sept.
CHPPD	6.1	6.2	5.9	6.0	5.9	5.9	5.8	5.8	5.7	5.5	7.0	6.1

Unfortunately, the data, while helpful, do not indicate the whys or whats. Why did the CHPPD decrease in July? Did it result from patient acuity or a lack of staff? What happened in August? Was staff back from vacation and available for work, while the physicians were on vacation and not admitting? Or did patient acuity increase? Trend data are useful, but they do not indicate the reasons for the trends, nor do they indicate the appropriate level to be attained.

It should also be noted that, while many ratios provide information that is interesting, they may not be indicative of productivity performance. For productivity-tracking purposes, a ratio showing worked hours per surgical case provides more relevant information than room minutes per surgical case.

The steps in establishing a ratio-trending system are relatively easy:

1. Determine the ratios to be monitored.
2. Establish the sources of data.
3. Develop the reporting procedure and related responsibilities.
4. Report the appropriate data.
5. Monitor the results.

This type of system, because of its simplicity, is a good starting point for performance tracking. The calculations are simple enough to allow for manual calculation on a timely basis.

With a monitoring system in place, management can begin to track the impacts on performance and productivity resulting from the changes implemented. By monitoring, organizations can determine whether desired results are being obtained.

Linkage with Compensation

The final and perhaps the most important management system to review is the compensation of line managers. The line manager (for example, the chief technologist, head nurse, or lead housekeeper) interprets for the staff the organization's productivity/efficiency strategy and ensures that it is carried out. Organizations have traditionally compensated all head nurses, for example, at essentially the same level, with minor variations for longevity, seniority, or education. Under the traditional system, maintaining the status quo is often the best route for employees to obtain salary increases.

By refocusing the reward mechanisms in order to compensate line managers according to the productivity, efficiency, and quality of their work, line managers become a conduit to change rather than a bottleneck. New skills and techniques are more readily assimilated when endorsed by line managers.

Such refocusing is never easy. Performance evaluation practices often have to be revised and objective performance expectations established. Position descriptions may have to be revised to address the new mandates placed on managers.

Managers are responsible for producing the services provided and managing the resource consumption associated with the output. The manager who produces the desired results with reduced inputs and maintains or improves quality is worth more to the organization than a manager who preserves the status quo.

Summary

Sustained productivity improvement is the product of the work of managers who are committed to the process and who have the ability to respond in a constantly changing health care arena. Management systems that are attuned to the organization's productivity strategy are easier to implement. Only then can the organization have a logical and consistent approach to productivity.

It should be noted that productivity improvement is not a short-term, one-time effort. Nor is it a public relations gimmick or the responsibility of one individual, such as the management engineer or the cost accountant. Rather, to be effective, lasting productivity improvement must be an integral part of the organization's survival strategy. It must mesh with the marketing and competition strategies and be consistent with quality expectations.

Chapter 4

Staffing for High Productivity

John A. Page
Mark D. McDougall

In general, as a department improves the match between its staffing patterns and work load, the utilization of staff increases. This chapter shows how higher productivity can be achieved through the improved management of work load and staffing patterns. This chapter also provides an overview of how to measure work load, determine staffing requirements, and assess a department's utilization of staff and performance in comparison with other hospital departments.

Understanding What Productivity Is

In general terms, productivity is simply a measure of the relationship of work expended and output gained, that is, the work used to produce a unit of output. In a health care environment, productivity is often measured in terms such as hours per patient day or hours per procedure. Departmental productivity is typically determined by dividing the required (or standard) hours by the actual hours worked. The result is the percentage of time the staff was effectively utilized. Therefore, *productivity* might be more appropriately termed effective utilization of staff.

The goal of any attempt to increase productivity should be to work smarter, not harder. Simply increasing the rate at which workers function does not, in the long run, provide substantial increases in productivity. Such an approach to increasing productivity may also have undesirable side effects, such as reduced morale or lower quality of work. In the long run, these side effects can have disastrous consequences that outweigh any short-term productivity increase achieved. Therefore, a major objective of increasing productivity is to eliminate the obstacles that impede effective and efficient operation.

As one might expect, many factors influence the productivity of any particular group of workers. These factors include the quantity of products produced and the amount of resources consumed. For example, the productivity of food service workers (measured in terms of meals per hour) would be significantly influenced by the number of meals to be prepared as well as by such things as the level of automation, the use of assembly-line tray preparation, the use of a bulk food production system, and the percentage of convenience or premade food items used in the system. In the clinical laboratory and radiology departments, economies of scale, automated procedures, and use of alternative resources can significantly affect the productivity of the staff.

In order to reach the desired levels of productivity, it is necessary to review those factors affecting productivity. Two important factors are the adequacy of employee skills and the matching of skills needed for a particular job with the personnel most likely to have those skills. For example, it would not be desirable to utilize an employee to assist with surgical procedures unless that person was trained to perform such demanding tasks. It is also important to realize that using nursing staff to routinely complete unskilled tasks (such as filling patient water pitchers) may be equally ineffective. Routinely matching a worker's skills with the skills necessary to complete a particular job is essential to achieving a high level of productivity. However, one must also temper that view by acknowledging that, in general, completing some productive work (even if the skills required are at a lower level than the skills possessed) is more desirable than remaining idle. In this case, if freeing up the nurses' time would result in the nursing personnel remaining idle and performing no activities while other workers performed such tasks, then having nurses perform unskilled tasks might be preferable.

To see how matching certain skills more effectively with the needs of the job can free up employees' time, let us examine the experience of a hypothetical radiology department. Let us further suppose that this department originally required each of the three radiology technicians to transport patients scheduled for examinations. Such transport activities constituted one-third of all technician hours worked. The three technicians each worked 1,000 hours to produce a department total of 3,000 examinations during one particular period of time. The amount of time worked by a technician was 1.00 hour per examination (3,000 hours worked [3 employees × 1,000 hours each] divided by 3,000 examinations performed).

To raise productivity, let us suppose that the radiology department administrator decided to hire a transport aide, who was required to work the same number of hours as each of the technicians. However, when patient volume in this hypothetical department remained constant during the time period of equal length that followed the hiring of the aide, the administrator found that having the additional staff member on board simply led to a reduction in productivity, for more resources were now being consumed to produce the same volume. The required time rose to 1.33 hours worked per examination (4,000 hours worked [4 employees × 1,000 hours each] divided by 3,000 examinations performed).

If the volume for this department had increased to 4,500 examinations during that time period, the radiology department administrator would have achieved the goal of increased productivity, with a required time of 0.88 hours worked per examination. In addition, if one assumes that the labor cost associated with the transport aide is less than that associated with the technician, an even greater increase in departmental productivity would have been achieved because less-costly resources (transport aide labor) would have been used. The administrator could have improved the productivity of the department, but success depended on the degree to which the technicians used their freed-up time to increase the volume of examinations.

Workers' attitudes are another important factor in achieving high levels of productivity. Motivated workers with a positive attitude toward their jobs are important to the productivity equation. Organizing and directing workers effectively also contributes to achieving and maintaining high levels of productivity.

In addition, organizing the work itself so that it is completed in the most effective manner can provide substantial increases in the overall productivity of any department. One facet of organizing the work involves the functional planning and layout of the workplace. Eliminating unnecessary travel or movement, appropriately sequencing tasks performed, and eliminating bottlenecks are also means by which productivity can be improved. Maintaining proper environmental conditions (such as lighting, temperature, and ventilation) are also important factors to be considered when providing a productive workplace. Finally, in order to accurately gauge the success of any attempts to improve productivity, adequate measures of work must be developed and maintained.

Following the Systems Approach to Productivity Improvement

Productivity improvement is more than just cutting staffing levels. There is no doubt that productivity can be improved by reducing the resources used in producing any given volume of work. However, productivity can also be improved by doing more with the same resources, by doing less with a proportionately greater reduction in resources used, or by doing more with a proportionately smaller increase in resources consumed.

Because health care organizations are increasingly emphasizing becoming lean and mean in the newly competitive health care market, the use of management engineering departments and systems professionals has become more widespread. The management engineer usually acts as an unbiased outside observer with a big-picture viewpoint (the ability to identify the impact of events on the system or the organization as a whole).

Steps in the Systems Approach

Just how does a systems professional identify and work toward solutions to operational problems in health care that inhibit high productivity? Typically, a methodical, logical approach is taken in reviewing the system and the interactions of its components. This approach, usually referred to as *the systems approach,* involves the following steps in uncovering and analyzing operational problems:

1. Define the question, such as, "Are we appropriately staffed in radiology?"
2. Define the problem, such as, "Current expenses in radiology exceed revenue by several thousand dollars."
3. Establish the method for studying the problem.
4. Anticipate the results of the study.
5. Evaluate the costs and benefits of the study and approach.
6. Perform the appropriate study.
7. Redefine problem and solution parameters.
8. Define alternative solutions.
9. Test alternatives (feasibility and cost/benefit).
10. Present findings.
11. Sell alternatives.
12. Implement the program.
13. Follow up on performance.

Achieving Higher Productivity

To improve operational efficiency and increase productivity, managers must gain a thorough understanding of the operation in question because knowing the operation or department is essential to being able to identify appropriate solutions to productivity questions. Having answers to basic operational questions is an essential starting point for any review.

One way to understand how a department operates is to discuss the operation with those individuals who work in the department on a daily basis. It is also wise to realize that the operation described in a department's policies and procedures manual may have little resemblance to the actual, day-to-day operation of the department. For this reason, it is extremely important to actually spend time in the department to review the processes by which the work is completed, observe the interaction of personnel and flow of work, and get a feel for the true operation and the players involved.

Beyond the value of the firsthand knowledge and understanding obtained through this approach, the approach can provide other secondary benefits, such as improved department acceptance of recommendations made and the public relations value of understanding the people who might be affected by changes in operations.

It is also essential for managers to identify (and quantify as much as possible) past and future programmatic changes. What did the addition of a new oncologist to the medical staff do to the hospital's volume? What will the new emphasis on rehabilitation do to the patient mix? Reviewing historical data can sometimes provide clues to what changes can be expected. By planning for those programmatic changes in advance, increases in productivity can be obtained.

Furthermore, managers must identify potential problem and focus areas early in the review process in order to ensure the ultimate success of a project. Several areas of possible problems that should routinely be considered when trying to increase departmental productivity include interdepartmental relationships, fluctuations in work load volume, work load scheduling, skill mix, and staffing patterns.

Interdepartmental Relationships

Health care delivery does not occur in a vacuum but requires the interaction of many departments and personnel. Identifying interdepartmental relationships can provide many opportunities for maximizing the productivity of the organization as a whole as well as the productivity of individual departments. Many managers fail to recognize that what they do in their departments often affects other departments.

For example, one intensive care nursing manager made the decision that a manual request form be used routinely for patients receiving a particular laboratory test. The decision was made in order to "improve the productivity of the unit clerks" because they "didn't have the time" to enter the patient information that was required when they requested the procedure through the hospital information system. This situation was tolerated because it seemed easier to accommodate this routine than to deal with the real problem and correct it. The laboratory technologist was then required to enter the data himself, which usually required at least one call to the nursing unit to obtain the missing patient information.

In the end, the overall cost of this "productivity improvement" to the whole organization, as well as to each department, was significantly higher than the initial automated entry process. Such a ripple effect can sometimes be significant and must be considered when proposed changes in operations are made. Hospitals are under increased pressure to reduce patient length of stay. Because departments are all competing for limited patient time in scheduling examinations, there will be more pressure to schedule and sequence patient procedures and examinations. This will require interaction and coordination by all hospital departments.

Fluctuations in Work Load Volume

Departments often follow distinct volume fluctuation patterns. In many cases, seasonal demand fluctuations or other fluctuations in activity levels lead to department-level peaks and valleys that can significantly affect productivity. For example, one operating room was affected significantly by the practice patterns of three surgeons. These three surgeons were avid hunters and invariably went on vacation during the first week of hunting season. Their absence led to a significant decrease in productivity for the OR staff, who had not adjusted staffing to accommodate this fairly predictable volume valley. Other types of volume fluctuations (by time of day or day of week or by month or season) can also influence departmental productivity and should always be considered.

Work Load Scheduling

The degree to which work load can be managed through scheduling is an important consideration in improving departmental productivity. Although some activities in the health care setting do occur with more randomness (such as emergency department visits) than others (such as scheduled elective surgery procedures), the increased ability of a department to schedule its activities and provide a more steady work load can provide significant improvements to productivity.

Changing the method of scheduling procedures can improve productivity. An example of this might be opening surgical schedule blocks 24 hours rather than 12 hours before the scheduled start time. This would help to accommodate increased use of available operating room time and reduce the impact of an unpredictable add-on schedule. Work load leveling, that is, eliminating the peak/valley syndrome typically associated with health care services, can be achieved through the increased use and sophistication of departmental work load scheduling.

Skill Mix

The skill mix of the staff is an important consideration in understanding how staffing affects productivity. Are the right people routinely available to complete the work to be done? Having the appropriate number of persons available to perform the work load says little about the ability of those persons to meet the given volume demand. For example, using 15 nurse's aides to accommodate the 15 full-time equivalent (FTE) requirements of a particular nursing unit obviously would be inappropriate. However, would the opposite (an all-RN staffing pattern) be considered inappropriate? Many institutions have taken pride in their all-RN staffs. But can that type of staffing be accommodated during an era of prospective pricing and nursing shortages? Probably not. Health care managers should look beyond the mentality that "an FTE is an FTE" and look at methods to better match activities with skills. In many cases, departments may be forced to analyze and update the job responsibilities of their current staff and make changes to provide the same (or even better) services at lower costs.

Staffing Patterns

A major goal of productivity improvement should also be to better match the available personnel resources with the work load to be completed. Work load usually does not fit smoothly into the typical 7-to-3 or 9-to-5 workday. By better accommodating inherent work load fluctuations (those that cannot be easily changed or scheduled), productivity improvements can be obtained.

In productivity improvement programs, all alternatives should be explored. One of the most fruitful areas that can be examined is the current staffing patterns within individual departments. Alternative staffing patterns and methods can provide more flexibility and increased efficiency and effectiveness in meeting departmental work load.

Several ideas should be considered. First, although hospitals seem obsessed with the concept of FTEs, they invariably consider hiring full-time personnel almost exclusively. In order to better accommodate a department's work load, the hospital might hire two (or more) part-time persons rather than one full-time person (2 × 0.5 FTE = 1.0 FTE). This is particularly useful in departments with uneven work loads, such as in diagnostic radiology, which traditionally has a higher early morning work load. Utilizing part-time personnel may also allow managers to implement flexible staffing (to better accommodate fluctuations in work load) and to allow for the hiring of personnel who have previously left the work force (for example, new mothers). Such personnel may not wish full-time employment, but their desired schedule may match work load peaks within the department.

Another concept that should be considered is utilization of floating personnel—personnel from a centralized float pool, temporary/registry personnel (such as those who have been used in nursing departments for years), or cross-trained personnel from other departments. Although obviously limited by the skills of the personnel available, cross-training can successfully provide increased productivity for the departments involved as well as an opportunity for more job satisfaction and expanded roles for the employee.

Also to be considered is flexible and staggered staffing patterns to move away from the traditional 7 a.m.–3 p.m., 3 p.m.–11 p.m., and 11 p.m.–7 a.m. schedules. Although moving away from such traditional schedules is sometimes difficult, alternative patterns may be more suited to a particular department's work load. For example, a clinic traditionally scheduled all personnel to start at 7:30 a.m., although the first patient was never scheduled before 8:45 a.m. In theory, this time was to be used for catching up, opening the clinic, and preparing for the day's schedule. In reality, only one nurse and one technologist were needed to handle these activities, and the remaining staff were essentially unproductive until the physicians appeared in the clinic (routinely not before 9 a.m.). In addition, afternoon clinics usually ran late, with the department incurring overtime and decreased morale because of constant unpredictability of schedules. In this case, one immediate solution was instituted—having the staff report at staggered times, with most scheduled to begin work between 8:30 a.m. and 9:00 a.m. The result was an immediate increase in productivity in addition to reduced overtime, improved morale, and the possibility of extending current clinic operating hours with the existing staff.

Other alternative staffing patterns include longer workdays (such as four 10-hour days per week or three 12-hour days for 40 hours' pay) or different shifts on different days (to better accommodate fluctuating work load patterns throughout the week). Innovative scheduling mechanisms such as these also improve staff morale. For example, a work week of four 10-hour days (even on a rotating basis) would give employees a three-day weekend every other week. Employing a different scheduling method (such as cyclical scheduling where predetermined scheduling patterns are identified and followed) and using computerized scheduling systems (which attempt to optimize scheduling patterns) should be options that are at least examined for feasibility.

The department's effectiveness in managing staff benefit time (such as education and vacation time) and the levels of other nonproductive time (such as sick hours or even daily break time) should also be considered. Significant losses in productivity can be tied to poor management or abuses in the use of employee benefit time. For example, encouraging (or requiring) employees to schedule vacation time during traditionally slow periods can provide increases in productivity by better matching personnel with resources necessary. In the OR example cited previously, encouraging employees to schedule vacation time during the hunting season when physicians were on vacation could add significantly to overall departmental productivity.

Also consider expanding the role certain staff members play. For example, it might be possible to train clinic technicians to routinely obtain patients' weight, temperature, and blood pressure when they place patients in examination rooms, thereby increasing the role the technicians play in the delivery of care as well as reducing the routine duties of the nursing staff.

Planning for Change

In order for things in any organization to change (and increasing productivity obviously involves some degree of change), management and non-management personnel must become involved in the process and work toward change. It is natural to resist change: A known is always easier to accept than an unknown. Therefore, in order to effectively initiate change, an attitude for change must be cultivated. Human nature tells us that part of the psychology of change should always include the education of and participation by those individuals affected by the change. Using a participative approach can establish the basis for accepting the productivity measures developed. Through their participation, the employees of a department buy into the measures from the beginning and feel a greater degree of ownership of the results.

Creativity and the use of nontraditional ideas are sometimes difficult to sell in an environment resistant to change. It is ironic that in medicine, a field undoubtedly experiencing constant change and growth, people sometimes resist changing the fundamental methods by which they accomplish (and even manage) the services they provide. Analyzing the factors that affect staffing (such as physician practice and ordering patterns), work flows or patient flows or both, and scheduling patterns can be important to developing alternatives through which productivity can be improved along with the quality of the services provided or the level of client satisfaction.

Encouraging an environment conducive to change is important to the ultimate success of any operations improvement. Although the impact of change on upper-level management may be minimal in most cases, an innovative and change-oriented environment must be cultivated from the top down. Such support may include the recognition or reward of personnel involved in successful change as well as the inclusion of goals in the organization's strategic plan that identify desired changes.

Equally important to successful operations improvement is the bottom-up support of the personnel most intimately involved with and affected by the change. At best, effecting change in any organization is difficult. It becomes much more difficult to implement, however, when it is imposed by others. Clearly, education and participation are the most important concepts in cultivating bottom-up change.

Another essential component of successful change is a thorough understanding of the existing system, identifying its strengths and weaknesses and determining whether the need for change is apparent. This understanding will help in estimating the impact of change and in identifying alternative methods.

Human nature does not make change easy. Dealing with the "we've always done it that way" attitude is an important barrier to overcome in any improvement project. One rule that should always be followed is to ask why: Why is an activity done? Why is it done that way? Why is it done by those personnel? Why is it done in that area? Questioning the why, what, when, where, who, and how of any operation is the single most important function in successfully identifying areas for change.

The use of process charts or flowcharts of the operation can assist in illustrating the inefficiencies inherent in any operation. Once again, one aspect of planning that cannot be emphasized enough is good communication and feedback to and from the personnel involved in an operation. Communication is important for adequately identifying areas for improvement and for anticipating the potential impact of the change to the department as well as to the organization as a whole.

As we have discussed, there are several keys to successfully implementing change in any organization. There is no magic formula for successful change. If anything, the keys to success seem to be common sense and intuition. That is the case with the following suggestions:

- Anticipate change.
- Plan for change.
- Start with an area with good potential for success.
- Weigh the costs and benefits of change.
- Involve employees throughout the process.
- Communicate, communicate, communicate.
- Avoid rapid change.
- Monitor and nurture behavioral changes.

Some general ideas for improvement that should always be considered include:

- Eliminating the activity altogether
- Combining activities
- Changing the sequence of activities
- Changing the location(s) where activities take place
- Changing the personnel completing the activities

Developing Labor Standards for Productivity Improvement

To assess utilization of staff and departmental performance, managers must first develop labor standards. A *labor standard* is the length of time required by staff to complete a certain activity. Three steps should be followed when developing labor standards to ensure their reliability and acceptance among department personnel:

1. Identify/define the activities performed in the department.
2. Select the activities that will serve as the work load indicators. A *work load indicator* is the unit of work load that is being measured, such as a chest X ray.

Identifying and Defining the Department's Activities

The first step in developing departmental labor standards is identifying the activities performed in the department. Accurately documenting those activities is essential to the development of accurate and reliable labor standards. Complete documentation also provides a detailed definition of the actions and tasks included in each defined activity. Definitions of what constitutes any given activity may vary from institution to institution or even among personnel within any given department. Proper and complete identification and documentation eliminates the possibility of misinterpreting the data and will improve the usability of the data developed in subsequent reviews.

Documentation of activities can be accomplished through various methods including narrative descriptions, activities flowcharting, and process charts. Although any method of documentation may be used, a combination of these three can provide a sufficiently detailed record of the activities performed. Also, although flow- and process charting are somewhat more difficult to learn and complete than narrative descriptions, the resulting illustrations of the system can be more helpful in understanding the activities of the department and identifying operational inefficiencies and bottlenecks. A sample flowchart for a medical records department correspondence clerk is provided in figure 4-1.

As part of the definition process, a department's activities can be classified into two categories: variable and fixed. Variable activities are those that fluctuate because of changing volumes. In a radiology department, variable activities include chest X rays, mammograms, X rays of the lower gastrointestinal tract, and the like.

Fixed (or constant) activities are activities that are essentially unaffected by fluctuations in patient volume. These activities include code cart checks, annual inventory, administrative meeting time, and personnel education and in-service functions. As one might imagine, these activities are not directly affected by patient volume fluctuations and remain constant, at least within a relative range. This relative range can be illustrated as a step function (figure 4-2).

Activities within each category may also be classified as direct (patient care activities) or indirect (support activities performed by department personnel). For example, direct variable activities include procedures performed on the patient, whereas indirect variable activities include scheduling, patient transport, billing and filing, and other activities associated with patient volumes. Managers need to take indirect activities into account when the time comes to determine the size of the required staff (this is discussed later).

Selecting Work Load Indicators

Once the department's activities have been identified and defined, appropriate work load indicators must be selected. These indicators must be

Figure 4-1. Sample Flowchart for a Medical Records Department Correspondence Clerk

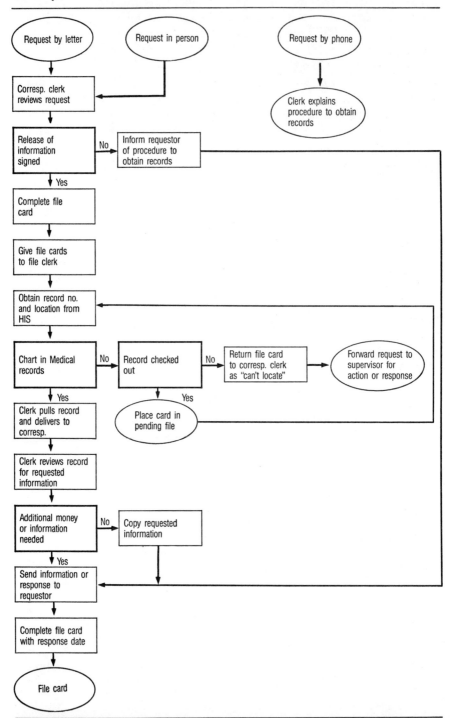

Figure 4-2. Direct and Indirect Staffing Needs

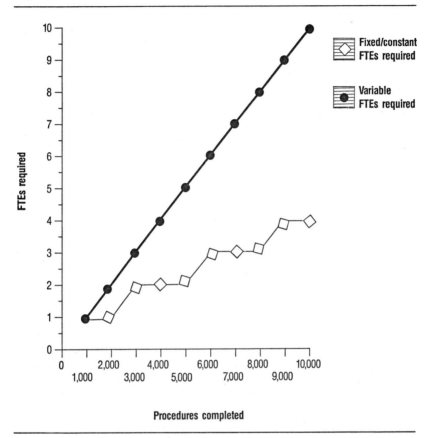

quantifiable and must give a good indication of the entire work load within the department. The level of detail necessary varies from department to department. Some departments may require a significant number of work load indicators to adequately determine their work load; others can use fewer indicators. It should be understood, however, that the greater the detail desired for measuring work load, the greater the effort will be to develop labor standards and the greater the commitment will be to continually gather the needed data.

For example, the radiology department of Hospital A has determined that detailed, procedure-level labor standards are necessary to adequately determine its constantly changing work load. Hence, this department uses numerous work load indicators in measuring its work load. Hospital B's radiology department, on the other hand, believes that it has a somewhat more consistent procedure mix and has decided that developing labor standards only on categories of procedures (such as within CPT coding categories: skull, abdomen, contrast G.I., and so forth) is appropriate and adequate to determine its work load. Hospital C's radiology department performs fairly routine radiology examinations without much fluctuation in the mix of examinations. This department believes that, for its use, a work load indicator such as X ray procedures, without further differentiation, is appropriate and adequate. As one might imagine, the methods of determining work load are as varied as the departments that will use them, and none of these three departments has chosen the only way.

When choosing work load indicators, the following considerations should be taken into account. First, hospitals should use the 80/20 approach by choosing work load indicators from the 20 percent of department activities that account for 80 percent of the volume. It is more important to have good and accurate measures on high-volume activities than to have less-than-accurate measures on all activities. (For example, a procedure that is only performed once per month in a laboratory would not be a good indicator of work load.) When determining volumes for department activities, managers will find that some volume data are more easily obtained than others, such as those that can be provided by the hospital billing system. In such cases, direct variable activities such as radiology procedures may be utilized as work load indicators.

It is not unusual, however, for a department to think that the charge codes used in the current billing system do not adequately define the work load within the department. This may be because the charge codes do not adequately differentiate between various procedures with respect to the levels of resources required or because the definitions are unclear or outdated. The hospital has the choice of either updating the charge codes or looking for alternative ways of measuring work load.

A second consideration in choosing work load indicators is that measuring individual work load (and therefore individual productivity) in a health care setting is difficult and estimated at best. Health care is unlike a manufacturing environment, where personnel complete a more narrow and discrete set of activities. For this reason, defining the work load or measuring the productivity of individuals becomes a much more difficult job. Department-level or cost-center-level productivity monitoring is usually the preferred method.

Developing Labor Standards

Labor standards provide a detailed and accurate measure of the time required to complete a given examination or procedure in a specific institution. There are many methods for developing labor standards, such as work sampling, in which random observations of workers are made to estimate the proportions of the workday being spent on various activities. Another is self-reporting/diaries, in which the workers themselves are asked to log the amounts of time they spend at various tasks. Both of these methods can estimate, over a specified period of time, the total hours utilized for specific activities that have been designated as work load indicators. These estimates should include only those hours actually worked. Unproductive hours, such as those for vacation, holidays, sick leave, and so forth, should not be included.

Once the total hours have been estimated for a particular activity, they are divided by the volume of activity during that specified period of time. The result is a labor standard. For example, if a department determined that 2,700 hours were worked to perform 1,000 EKGs in the past year, the labor standard could be 2.7 hours worked per EKG performed (2,700 divided by 1,000). An alternative to performing calculations such as this is to use "canned" labor standards, or preestablished industry standards, rather than having the hospital determine standards for itself.

Another alternative for developing labor standards is participative analysis, a form of which is to bring staff members of a department together as an expert group that has daily, firsthand knowledge of the activities performed in the department. Known as the Delphi approach, this process aims at achieving a consensus on what the labor standards should be. The Delphi approach can be time-consuming but has improved the long-term benefits of the productivity program by increasing department understanding and acceptance as well as by improving the accuracy of the results obtained.

Whatever labor standards are developed, managers must ensure that they are updated as necessary in order to maintain their integrity. Only labor standards that are accurate can be utilized as a starting point in staffing for productivity improvement.

Determining Utilization Targets

Once the labor standards have been established for the work load indicators in a department, the department needs to determine a desired target for the utilization of its staff before it can assess its staff utilization and performance. Established targets express in percentages the desired match between staff and work load. For example, a department with a utilization target of 80 percent is expected to have some unproductive staff time owing to uncontrollable or less controllable operational factors (table 4-1).

Although identifying operational factors that affect the utilization of staff may be relatively easy, determining an exact utilization target is not. Nonetheless, three possible methods of approximating appropriate utilization targets are the following:

- Review historical (actual) levels of utilization among management engineering, department management, and hospital administration personnel and negotiate an appropriate utilization target.
- Quantify all delays and downtime, rectify the avoidable delays, and establish the utilization target on the basis of the unavoidable delays

Table 4-1. Factors Affecting Staff Utilization

Controllable	Uncontrollable or Less Controllable
• Scheduling of staff • Easily scheduled work load • Prioritizing work load and postponing deferrable work load to slower periods in shift, day, week, month, and year • Avoidable delays • Scheduling of vacations • Job sharing (intradepartmental and interdepartmental) • Reducing downtime by sending employees home early when work load permits (if policy allowed/required such action)	• Substantial work load fluctuations throughout day, shift, week, month, and year • Unavoidable delays • Physician ordering patterns • Stat orders • Quality of service expectations (for example, turnaround time and waiting time) • Sick leave • Market constraints regarding the availability and use of part-time positions for improving the match between staff and work load

and acceptable levels of downtime (for example, minimal staffing requirements for providing acceptable levels of service).

- Calculate an overall weighted average utilization target on the basis of the distribution of work load by shift and the accepted utilization levels by shift (or portion thereof). This calculation is done by multiplying the percentages of work load for each shift by the percentages of expected utilization. An example of this method, representing a radiology department's typical heavy morning work load, is provided in table 4-2.

Establishing a utilization target for any department quantifies the expected performance of that department by management/administration. Factors specific to particular departments are difficult to generalize. For overall reference, table 4-3 provides a listing of typical departmental utilization targets. The values provided are those that might be expected in a typical department and should be used for overall guidance in establishing utilization targets.

Determining the Size of the Required Staff

The next step in assessing both utilization of staff and departmental performance is determining the total number of paid FTEs required by a department to handle the anticipated work load. This number is computed as follows:

Add together the volumes for the variable activities (work load indicators) to determine the total activities (referred to henceforth as *procedures*).

Table 4-2. Weighted Average Utilization Target for a Radiology Department, Based on Work Load Fluctuations by Shift

Shift	Percent of Work Load (1)	Expected Utilization (Percent) (2)	Weighted Utilization (1 × 2)
Morning	40	95	0.380
Afternoon	20	65	0.130
Evening	30	75	0.225
Night	10	50	0.050
Total	100		0.785

Weighted average utilization target 78.5%

Table 4-3. Typical Utilization Targets for Hospital Departments

Department	Typical Utilization Target
Ancillary Services	
Electrocardiology	80–95%
Electroencephalography	80–95%
Laboratory	80–95%
Pharmacy	80–95%
Physical therapy	80–95%
Radiology	70–95%
Respiratory therapy	80–95%
Nursing Services	
Critical care	75–95%
Emergency room	60–90%
Labor and delivery	40–80%
Medical/surgical unit	90–100%
Nursery	70–90%
Obstetrics	75–95%
Operating room	70–95%
Pediatrics	75–95%
Recovery room	70–90%
Support Services	
Administration	85–100%
Admitting	75–95%
Business office	90–100%
Central supply	85–100%
Communications	90–100%
Data processing	90–100%
Dietary/food services	85–100%
Education	85–100%
Fiscal services	85–100%
Housekeeping	85–100%
Laundry and linen	85–100%
Maintenance	85–100%
Management engineering	85–100%
Medical records	85–100%
Personnel	90–100%
Security	90–100%
Social services	90–100%

The result is Quantity A. (Table 4-4 provides an example of this and subsequent calculations described in the following paragraphs.)

Next, multiply the volume for each procedure over a given period by the labor standard for each procedure to determine the standard hours for each procedure for the period. Then add all the standard hours together. This sum is the direct procedure hours (Quantity B).

Next, determine the estimated time spent on indirect (or support) activities for the procedures (an example of which is shown in table 4-5). Multiply this estimated time by Quantity A to compute the total indirect (support) hours (Quantity C).

Table 4-4. Example of a Technologist and Management Staffing Analysis for Diagnostic Radiology

Variable Activities (procedures designated as work load indicators)	Volume (no. of procedures per 30-day period)	Labor Standard (hours per exam)	Standard Hours for 30-Day Period
Abdomen	226	0.24	54.24
Angioplasty	1	3.00	3.00
Chest/ribs	2717	0.18	489.06
Esophagus	46	0.35	16.10
Gallbladder	63	0.58	36.54
Head/neck	336	0.33	110.88
I.V.P.	201	1.15	231.15
Lower extremity	772	0.26	200.72
Lower G.I.	179	0.74	132.46
Mammogram	536	0.58	310.88
Portable	675	0.13	87.75
	5752		1672.78

Total volume of activities (procedures) (A)	A = 5752
Total direct procedure hours (B)	B = 1672.78
Indirect (support) hours (C) = 0.25 × (A) (at 0.25 hours per procedure in this example)	C = 1438.00
Subtotal variable hours required (D) = (B) + (C)	D = 3110.78
Department utilization target (E) (in this example)	E = 78.50%
Total variable hours required (normalized) (F) = $\frac{(D)}{(E)}$	F = 3962.78
Constant hours (G) (30 days at 24.32 hours per calendar day [in this example])	G = 729.60
Total target worked hours required (H) = (F) + (G)	H = 4692.38
Total target FTEs required (I) = (H) divided by 173.33 (hours per FTE per month)	I = 27.07 FTEs
Vacation/holiday/sick FTE allowance (J) = (I) × 12.5% [percentage varies by hospital department]	J = 3.38 FTEs
Total required paid FTEs (K) = (I) + (J)	K = 30.45 FTEs

Table 4-5. Quantification of Indirect (Support) Activity in One Radiology Department

Indirect Activity	Minutes per Occurrence	Frequency per Examination	Allocated Time per Examination (minutes × frequency)
Examination scheduling	1.5	1.0	1.5
Patient transport (round trip)	15.0	.5	7.5
File clerk	2.5	2.0	5.0
Darkroom/quality control	2.0	1.0	2.0
Report transcription	3.5	1.0	3.5
Total support time per examination (in minutes)			19.50

Add Quantity B to Quantity C to determine the subtotal variable hours required (Quantity D).

Determine the utilization target (Quantity E) for the department (as explained in the last section).

Divide Quantity D by Quantity E to compute the total variable hours required. This total is *normalized,* meaning that it is made on the basis of a utilization target of 100 percent for purposes of being able to compare staff requirements of one department with those of other departments in the hospital.

Next, add up the number of staff hours spent per day in fixed activities, such as meetings, classes, inventories, and so forth. Multiply this number by the number of days in the period under study. The result is the total number of hours of fixed activity, or *constant hours* (Quantity G), in the period.

Add Quantity F to Quantity G to compute the total target worked hours required (Quantity H).

Divide Quantity H by 173.33 (hours per FTE per month) to compute the total target FTEs required (Quantity I).

Multiply Quantity I by the percentage of paid staff time in the department for vacation, holidays, and sick leave. The result is the vacation/holiday/sick-leave FTE allowance (Quantity J, in FTEs).

Add Quantity I to Quantity J to determine the total required paid FTEs.

Assessing Utilization of Staff and Departmental Performance

Once the utilization target and total required paid FTEs have been determined, managers are in a position to assess both the department's utilization of staff and its performance in comparison with other hospital departments. Utilization of staff is calculated by using the following equation:

$$\text{Utilization of Staff} = \frac{\text{Required Staff (in FTEs)}}{\text{Actual Staff (in FTEs)}}$$

The result of that calculation can be plugged into another equation to determine *normalized performance,* a figure that allows managers to compare the performance of one department with that of another. Normalized performance values are made on the basis of an organizationwide utilization target of 100 percent as a common comparison base. Normalized performance is computed as follows:

$$\text{Normalized Performance} = \frac{\text{Utilization of Staff}}{\text{Department Utilization Target}}$$

In addition to performing these calculations, managers should establish an acceptable operating range using the department utilization target as a midpoint. This range provides the acceptable boundaries of performance for the department and clearly defines performance expectations in advance.

As an example of computing both utilization of staff and normalized performance, a study in a hypothetical diagnostic radiology department might have determined the following:

Required staff = 22.5 FTEs (at 100% utilization)

Actual staff = 29.8 FTEs

Department utilization target = 78.5%

Acceptable range of performance = Target plus or minus 5%

$$\text{Utilization of staff} = \frac{22.5}{29.8} = 0.755 = 75.5\%$$

$$\text{Normalized performance} = \frac{0.755}{0.785} = 0.962 = 96.2\%$$

In this example, the utilization of staff was below the utilization target of 78.5 percent but within the department's acceptable range of performance of 73.5 percent to 83.5 percent (or 78.5 percent plus or minus 5 percent). Therefore, the utilization of staff within the radiology department for the period was acceptable.

In comparison with other hospital departments, the normalized performance was also acceptable. The normalized acceptable range of performance for this hypothetical department is 95 percent to 105 percent (or 100 percent [the common comparison base] plus or minus 5 percent). The value of 96.2 percent determined here easily falls within that range.

Using Productivity Monitoring and Reporting Systems

Developing accurate and appropriate productivity measures is futile without developing appropriate mechanisms to monitor and report department productivity. A productivity monitoring and reporting system is one component of an overall hospital management information system and is a method for tracking and evaluating the effectiveness of labor utilization over time. Typical objectives of a productivity monitoring and reporting system include:

- Providing department managers and administrators with periodic reports of labor utilization and departmental performance
- Monitoring the attainment of departmental productivity goals and targets
- Collecting and summarizing the data to be utilized in the planning and budgeting of resources
- Providing timely information that can be used to justify costs, budgets, and reimbursements
- Aiding the evaluation of the impact of new equipment, services, policies, and procedures or regulations on services or resources
- Providing an indicator of those areas where costs can be reduced, thereby contributing to the overall organizational goal of cost containment

A *productivity monitoring and reporting system,* then, is a mechanism to report the utilization of staff in a manner that allows management and administration to identify operational fluctuations and make informed decisions.

Although productivity reports may contain many types of useful information, some types of information are essential:

- Actual work load volumes for the period
- Actual hours worked for the period
- Actual nonproductive hours paid for the period

Such data form the basis for informal decisions on staff utilization and enable managers to monitor their progress toward greater productivity.

Conclusion

Productivity monitoring and organizational productivity improvements are not isolated events and should be considered ongoing and essential components of an innovative and progressive organization. Incorporating productivity improvement into the organization's strategic plans is essential to maintaining a visible commitment to change on the part of senior-level and department-level managers alike.

Including productivity monitoring and improvement activities in departmental goals and objectives is also necessary in developing an effective action plan. As part of the formal goals of the department, department managers and hospital administrators should establish appropriate utilization targets and an acceptable range of performance. These goals should be realistic and achievable.

Continuous challenge is important to the success of any management program. Organizations must maintain the edge necessary to be leaders and hence must plan for continuous productivity improvement. Remember, as they say in dogsled racing, unless you are the lead dog, your view never changes.

Chapter 5

Productivity and Quality Management

John P. Werner

Introduction

Health care managers might claim that quality cannot be maintained or improved if resources are constrained or restricted. With the application of proper management techniques, however, quality and productivity can be improved at the same time. American automobile manufacturers used these techniques to respond to competition from the Japanese. A close relationship between quality and productivity has been proved in other industries, in manufacturing as well as in service industries such as banking and hotels. The objective of this chapter is to review some of the concepts and tools that are available to support managers in achieving productivity and quality.

The Effect of Quality Programs on Productivity

To discuss quality programs, one must first define the term *quality*. Although many prominent individuals within the health care field have had difficulty in developing a definition of quality, a simple definition will be used in this chapter: Quality is defined as meeting your customer's expectations.

As the following example shows, meeting your customer's expectations in Japan is a very serious, and sometimes literal, goal. In Japan the emphasis is on making it right the first time. This is the only way to efficiently produce a superior product.

In one instance, when IBM ordered a shipment of semiconductors from one of the better Japanese producers, the purchase contract specified that the acceptable defective rate of shipped product was three defective units out of 10,000 units produced. This was about as good as one could have expected from the best screening, after-the-fact sampling inspection plan. The Japanese producer was confused: The company intentionally made three defective items for each 10,000 good ones, put them in a separate package along with the shipment, and stated, "If you must have them, here they are." This company's process had been engineered and was subsequently so well controlled that it would make *no* defective units at all. But the Japanese producer wanted to meet their customer's expectation of three defective units out of 10,000 units produced (Gitlow and Gitlow, 1987).

Quality versus Capacity/Capabilities

Some may argue that the definition of quality as meeting your customer's expectations is too simple or perhaps even too complex. One problem in the health care field is that many health care managers confuse the word *quality* with *capacity/capabilities*. For example, when one reads in the press that reductions in health care expenditures will limit or decrease access to health care services and will thus compromise the quality of the services being provided, the issue actually being discussed is service capacity or service capabilities, not the quality of the services provided. Services will still be provided in accordance with acceptable clinical and service delivery standards. In some cases, however, these services may not use state-of-the-art technology; they may use older technology. Although older technology may not provide the same level of diagnostic information or the same degree of patient comfort, it would be used in accordance with acceptable standards, and the quality of the services provided would not be compromised.

For example, a patient could have kidney stones removed via surgery, that is, through older technology, or have them dissolved with a lithotripter, that is, through state-of-the-art technology. As far as the patient is concerned, the result may be the same, but the amount of discomfort, the level of clinical risk, the duration of the service encounter, and the cost of the services (and the revenue for the provider) will be different. The quality of care (defined as having met the customer's expectations) could be the same under both forms of technology.

The preceding discussion shows that quality and capacity/capability (that is, technology or the method for delivering the service) are not the same. This is also true in areas besides health care, for example, in the consumer product area. If a consumer's expectation is to acquire an automobile for personal transportation, the consumer could purchase a Chevrolet or a BMW. Either car would meet the expectation of the consumer, although one would cost three times as much as the other. The quality of both cars could fully meet the expectations of the consumer as well.

Relationship of Quality and Productivity

If we assume that this chapter's working definition of quality is valid, we can now explore the relationship between quality and productivity. To be objective, health care managers must discard the popular misconception that quality and productivity cannot be improved at the same time. This misconception is largely the byproduct of the cost-reimbursement era, better known as the "more is always better than less" era. Improvements in productivity are usually associated with improvements in quality. The following example will help to illustrate this relationship.

A study request was initiated by the director of the Medical Records Department of a 320-bed tertiary care teaching facility to investigate the charting of radiology reports in the patients' medical records. This request was presented to the facility's Management Engineering Department and was subsequently approved. By recording the number of reports that were received uncharted in the Medical Records Department, the director determined that the chart assembly clerks were charting 60 to 80 reports per week. These reports were being received by the department after patients had been discharged. This work load not only compromised the ability of the chart assemblers to complete their routine assignments, it also compromised the quality of the services provided to the patients. When the report was not available before a patient's discharge, either the attending physician would have to call the Radiology Department to obtain the results or the results of the radiology test would not be considered in making clinical decisions on the patient's treatment plan, including the discharge decision.

The results of the investigative study were as follows:

- The time required to process an order for a radiology examination (that is, from the time the physician wrote the order in the medical chart to the time that the results report was charted) had never been measured before at this hospital. The chairman of the Radiology Department stated upon inquiry that his standard for this statistic was 24 hours. However, when asked whether he had ever measured the capability of the current process, his response was, "No, but I know we average 24 hours."
- Compilation of statistics from existing records showed that the average time was 48 hours for examinations performed on Monday, Tuesday, Wednesday, or Thursday. When examinations were performed on Friday, Saturday, or Sunday, the average time increased to 72 hours.
- The charting of the reports by the radiology clerk was a full-time job on a Monday-through-Friday work schedule.
- The medical records chart assemblers worked an average of 20 hours per week in overtime to complete all of their assignments.
- Radiology physicians spent an average of one hour per day responding to telephone inquiries to provide results to attending physicians, results that were typed on the radiology reports.

After these results were reviewed with the appropriate individuals, the following recommendations were presented by the management engineer, discussed, and approved for implementation. The first recommendation was to develop and implement a quality control system to continuously monitor the charting process for radiology test results. The implementation of this system would require the radiology clerks to enter data, using a variables sampling plan, onto a standard process quality control record (figure 5-1). The data for this record were already available on the radiology report. This record contained daily sample data that were summarized every two weeks (one week's data are shown in figure 5-1). At the end of two weeks, the record was distributed to the director of medical records and to personnel within the Radiology Department.

A corresponding process was implemented in medical records to monitor the number of uncharted radiology reports and to report the results to appropriate personnel every two weeks. In this application, an attributes (acceptable or not acceptable, with an uncharted report classified as not acceptable) sampling program was used.

The second recommendation was that personnel work schedules within the transcription function should provide coverage on Saturday and Sunday. As stated earlier, if an examination was performed on Friday, Saturday, or Sunday, the charting of the report required an additional 24 hours. Upon investigation, the reason for this was obvious. The transcription function was not staffed on Saturday or Sunday. As expected, the transcription work load on Monday and Tuesday was much higher than it was for the remainder of the work week. Rather than hiring additional transcription clerks, the hospital revised the work schedules to provide service on Saturday and Sunday without any corresponding increase in the staffing requirements.

Providing service seven days rather than five days per week also had a beneficial impact on the charting process. Before these changes were implemented, finding a patient's medical record on the nursing unit was a common problem for the radiology clerk. The patient's location as entered on the radiology report was at least two to three days old by the time that the clerk arrived on a unit to chart the report. Given the nature of the services being provided at this hospital, patients were often transferred between nursing units. To investigate this problem, time studies were made on the basis of observations of the clerk's work routine. When these were completed, it was determined that, on average, the clerk spent two additional hours each workday locating patients who had been transferred.

After the need to improve the charting process became obvious, and the revised staffing schedules within the transcription function were implemented, the average time to chart a report was reduced from a range of 48 to 72 hours to an average of 30 hours. Within these time frames, the time that the radiology clerk spent locating transferred patients was reduced from 2 hours to 0.5 hours. This reduction made it possible to change the clerk's work schedule from a five-day schedule to a seven-day schedule to provide service coverage on Saturday and Sunday. The clerk's new work schedule was as follows:

Day of the Week	Work Schedule	Hours
Monday–Friday	7:00 a.m. to 1:30 p.m.	30
Saturday	7:00 a.m. to 11:00 a.m.	4
Sunday	7:00 a.m. to 11:00 a.m.	4
	Total per week	38

As shown, although the radiology clerk previously worked 40 hours per week, under the revised schedule, the clerk works only 38 hours per week. The clerk's hourly rate was adjusted so that the clerk still receives the same annual salary. This arrangement was implemented to reward the clerk for working a nonstandard work schedule. Because the clerk would now be working seven days a week, another clerk would work the above schedule every other week so that both clerks would be off every other weekend.

As a result of these changes, the overtime worked by the chart assemblers to chart uncharted radiology reports was eliminated, and the time spent by the radiologists on responding to telephone inquiries was reduced by 50 percent, from an average of 1 hour to 0.5 hours per day. The implementation of a quality performance measurement process as described resulted in many benefits; quality and productivity both improved at the same time (table 5-1).

The approach illustrated by the case example can be applied to many different situations with similar results. The next section of this chapter will further expand upon the techniques presented in this example.

Quality-Management Techniques

Before specific techniques are presented in this section, a conceptual framework will illustrate how the application of data collection and analysis techniques supports the quality objectives of the health care industry. It is important to understand how the services provided by one department relate to the services provided by another department and how all of these services relate to the customer's expectations during the patient care delivery process. It is easy to collect data; it is not always easy to collect the right data.

Recent Research in Quality Management

A recent article by Carol King (1987), entitled "A Framework for a Service Quality Assurance System," begins with some examples. In the service delivery world, the word *quality* is often still used as a value judgment meaning

Figure 5-1. Process Quality Control Record: Radiology Charting Process

Department-description	Number	Report maintained by
Radiology		J. Doe

Section A. Inspection Information

Date	4/6 Sun.	4/7 Mon.	4/8 Tues.	4/9 Wed.	4/10 Thu.	4/11 Fri.	4/12 Sat.
Medical record no.	704						
	728						
	801						
	745						
	301						
Inspected by	J.D.						
No. inspected/sample size (N)	5	5	5	5	5	5	5

Section B. Variable Measurement Results ($\bar{X}$)

Characteristic No.

#1 (Elapsed time (hours) from order written to result charted)	4/6	4/7	4/8	4/9	4/10	4/11	4/12	Total
	33	25						
	29	30						
	30	27						
	31	29						
	22	24						
No. of defects	145	135	155	160	155	150	150	1050
Average $\bar{x} = \frac{\Sigma x}{n}$	29	27	27	31	32	31	30	29.6

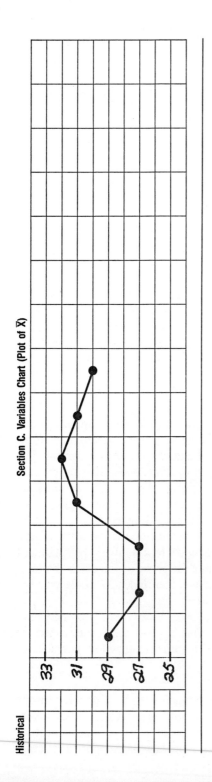

Table 5-1.   Benefits Summary: Radiology Report Charting Process

Quality Characteristics	(1) Before	(2) After	(3) = (1) − (2) Net Change
1. Examinations performed on Mon., Tue., Wed., or Thu.— Average charting time (hours)	48	30	(18)
2. Examinations performed on Fri., Sat., or Sun.— Average charting time (hours)	72	30	(42)
3. Medical records chart assemblers—overtime (hours/week)	20	0	(20)
4. Radiologists—telephone inquiry response time (hours/day)	1	0.5	(0.5)
5. Radiology clerk—charting time when patient location is incorrect (hours/day)	2	0.5	(1.5)
6. Radiology clerk—scheduled work hours (hours/week)	40	38	(2.0)

either good or bad; for example, "This is a quality outfit," "We sell a quality hot dog," and "We provide the highest quality health care." Along this line, fast food is usually considered to be of lower quality than food served in a high-priced French restaurant. But this line of thinking can be disastrous, as discovered by restaurateurs who introduced luxury restaurants into market areas where the customers wanted fast food. Again, it is important to determine your customer's expectations before you develop and establish new programs or services.

As a start, one can review the operational definition of quality assurance from the manufacturing world. Figure 5-2 provides a structural comparison between manufacturing and service industry quality programs. The manufacturing model starts with quality of design and identifies the product characteristics desired by the user. Standards are then established for those characteristics, and the product is designed to meet these standards. In production, conformance to standards is measured by testing or inspecting (measuring) the output, or both, and by monitoring the input (materials, labor skills, and so forth) and the production process itself. Nonstandard output (product) is analyzed to determine the cause of failure so that corrective actions can be taken. The process is then repeated to see whether the corrective actions were successful.

Leonard Berry and his coworkers (1985) at Texas A & M University have researched service quality from the customer's perspective. They asked the question: What is service quality? These researchers drew four conclusions from this study:

- Consumers' perceptions of service quality result from comparisons of their expectations before they receive the service to their actual experience with the service. Service quality is judged on the basis of whether or not it met expectations. Note how this supports the earlier

Figure 5-2. Structural Comparison of Manufacturing to Service Industries Quality Programs

Manufacturing Quality Control	Service Industries Quality Control	Behavioral Quality Control

Quality of Design:
• Define customer requirements
  —Identify desired quality characteristics
	Quality of Design:
	• Define customer wants and expectations
	  —Identify desired quality characteristics
	  —Define desired image
		Quality of Design:
		• Define customer needs and expectations
		  —Identify desired behaviors
		  —Determine the behavioral components of desired image
		• Define employee needs and expectations

Set product standards:
• Design product to meet those standards
  —Drawings
  —Raw product specs
  —Equipment specs
  —Production line design
	Set service levels:
	• Design service delivery and support systems
	  —Document the procedures
	  —"Plan B" procedures
	  —Space planning
	  —Equipment selection
	  —Specs for supplies
	  —Technical training
		Set behavioral guidelines:
		• Design the organization
		  —Interpersonal communication techniques
		  —Organizational values
		• Support Systems
		  —Recruitment
		  —Training
		  —Employee concerns
		  —Supervision

Quality of Conformance:
• Output measures:
  —Testing
  —Inspecting
• Process measures:
  —Raw product
  —Equipment monitoring
 	
• Combined measures:
 	
• When nonstandard output occurs:
  —Rework or scrap the rejects
  —Analyze rejects for cause of failures
  —Adjust production system
	Quality of Conformance:
	• Customer satisfaction measures:
	  —Customer complaint analysis
	  —Solicited customer feedback (comment cards, surveys)
	• Transaction observation
	• Shopping services
	  —Operating audits
	  —Operating statistics
	  —Technical training
	
	  —Peer review
	  —Research studies
	
	  —Make it right for the customer
	  —Determine cause
	  —Take corrective action
		Quality of Conformance:
		  —Customer complaints and solicited feedback
		  —Shopping services
		  —Transaction observation
		
		  —Employee morale measures
		  —Statistics—support services
		  —Operating audits of employee facilities
		  —Training—interpersonal and coping skills
		
		  —Make it right for the customer
		  —Determine cause
		  —Involve employees in problem solving

Source: King (1987). Reprinted, with permission, from *Quality Progress*, published by American Society for Quality Control, Copyright 1987.

definition of quality presented in this chapter (quality is defined as meeting your customer's expectations).

- Quality evaluations derive from the service process as well as from the service outcome. The way the service is performed can be a crucial component of the service from the consumer's point of view.
- Service quality is of two types. First, there is the quality level at which the regular service is delivered, such as a nurse's handling of a routine request from a patient. Second, there is the quality level at which exceptions or problems are handled, such as when a patient has been waiting in the Admissions Office for three hours for a bed assignment.
- When a problem occurs, the low-contact service firm becomes a high-contact service firm.

Berry's research focused only on the customer's perception of service quality. It did not consider the quality of the delivery processes that provide service to the consumer per se. The perspective of the customer is very important, but it may not be as important in the health care delivery process as the measurable quality of the delivery processes that provide care during a customer's service episode. Most health care consumers can determine whether the hotel services they need are provided in a high-quality manner: Is the food good? Is the room clean? Are the staff prompt and courteous? Was a bed available when promised? However, they usually cannot evaluate whether the clinical side of the delivery process is operating in a high-quality manner. Patients cannot determine whether the correct intravenous fluid is being administered or whether it is being administered at the correct flow rate.

A Systems Approach to Quality Management

In designing a quality-management program for a health care facility, not only should the hotel services side of the business be included, but the clinical or service delivery side also needs to be considered. When one designs a program, a systems approach can prove to be beneficial. A systems approach considers input (that is, resources such as labor, supplies, facilities, and equipment), the patient care delivery process, and the output produced by the process. For example, was the patient's health status improved; was the patient satisfied with the care provided by the process? The quality-management program measures and evaluates the use of the inputs in the process in order to respond to deficiencies in the output. The same approach, with some adaptations, can be used in designing a program at the facilitywide level or at the department/function level.

Taking the Initial Steps

The first thing a manager needs to do is to define what the patient's (customer's) expectations are, both from a hotel services standpoint and from a health care service delivery or outcome standpoint. Given these expectations, the next step is to review the process for the delivery of services and the inputs (labor skills, equipment, materials/supplies, facilities, operational systems, and so forth) that are required by the delivery process to provide the service. When completing this review, it may be a good idea to develop a flow diagram of the department (figure 5-3) or process (figure 5-4) under consideration.

Identifying Quality Performance Characteristics

Once the flow diagram has been prepared, quality performance characteristics should be identified for measurement purposes. Using the example illustrated in figure 5-4, the following characteristics could be selected:

- Elapsed time from request assigned to arrival at pickup area
- Elapsed time from arrival at pickup area to departure from pickup area

Figure 5-3. Department Flow Diagram: Direct Patient Care Department

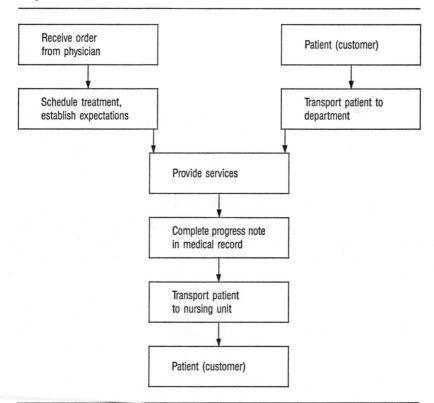

Figure 5-4. Process Flow Diagram: Patient Transport Department

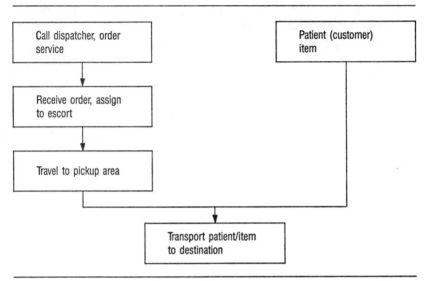

- Elapsed time from departure from the pickup area to arrival at destination area
- Number of assignment delays by probable cause (for example, escort not available, transportation equipment not available)
- Number of en route delays by probable cause (for example, elevator delays)
- Number of pickup area delays by probable cause (for example, lack of a wheelchair, lack of a stretcher, patient not ready, patient not available because he or she is receiving treatment in another department, specimen/document not available in the assigned pickup area)

Developing Instructions for Quality Inspections

After the characteristics have been selected for measurement, the procedure for conducting the quality inspections should be developed. The quality inspection instructions, as they are called in the manufacturing industry, usually detail the following:

- The sampling plan (for sample size selection instructions, see appendix A and table A-1).
- The inspection points (where and when inspections are to be conducted)
- The equipment (required measurement equipment is specified; for example, a scale to weigh a medication)
- The inspection record (the form or document on which the inspection results should be recorded)

- The reports (the form or report document that summarizes the results of the inspection measurements and, if applicable, the calculated sample statistics; for example, the mean, standard deviation, and range

[The book by Berger and Hart (1986) should be consulted when investigating the use and application of standard statistical quality-control techniques.] Examples of quality inspection instructions and report documents are illustrated in figure 5-1 and figure 5-5, which combines the sample size specification with the inspection record and report on the same form.

The example in figure 5-5 shows how the inspection specifications were adapted for application on the department level at an academic medical center. In this application, each quality characteristic or question is assigned to one of several characteristic categories. For example, the following categories are used at the medical center, with the definitions as noted:

- Procedural, includes characteristics/questions related to:
  - The patient's physical well-being or emotional needs
  - Procedural or service delivery technique
  - Omission or error in providing the service
- Service, includes characteristics/questions related to:
  - Timeliness of a response to a service request
  - Audit controls
  - Provision of hotel services
- Records/documentation, includes characteristics/questions related to:
  - Completeness
  - Correct entries
  - Control procedures
  - Problem identification
  - Follow-up action
- Equipment maintenance, includes characteristics/questions related to:
  - Calibration and preventive maintenance
  - Failure analysis and problem identification
  - Appearance/cleanliness
- Bacteriological measurements, includes characteristics/questions related to:
  - Sterility requirements
  - Response to infection control requirements
- Public relations, includes characteristics/questions related to:
  - Employee attitudes
  - Interdepartmental communications
  - Employee appearance or adherence to dress code requirements
- Area maintenance, includes characteristics/questions related to:
  - Adherence to housekeeping standards

Not all of these categories apply in every department, and in some cases other categories that are not listed may apply. The example in figure 5-5 does not use all seven categories. Individual characteristics or questions are assigned to a category so that a relative weight can be assigned to the category. These weights are then used to calculate a weighted quality score for each category. Table 5-2 provides an example of the calculation of the scores for each category. As shown in this example, category 5, bacteriological measurements, does not apply. The raw scores are calculated as follows:

$$\text{Raw Score} = \frac{\text{Total Number of "Yes" Responses for a Category}}{\text{Total Number of Observations Made} \times 100}$$

An example of a quality control report from the medical center is presented later in this chapter. This example will describe how the data presented in table 5-2 can be integrated into a useful management reporting system.

Key Strategies for Quality-Management Programs

As with any other program, ensuring the commitment of top-level management to quality-management programs is vital for the success of these programs. Because many top-level managers do not have previous experience with quality-management programs, obtaining their commitment will not be an easy task.

Top-Level Commitment

More health care executives should show their public commitment to quality with an adequate commitment of resources to support a viable program. Most acute care providers do not make an adequate investment in quality, which is not only an investment in management but in program support resources (staff, capital, and so forth). A review of the operating expense budgets at most major acute care providers would clearly support this

Table 5-2. Example of Calculation of Quality Scores

Category	(1) Relative Weight	(2) Raw Score	(3) = (1) × (2) Weighted Score
1. Procedural	20.0	85.0%	17.0
2. Service	20.0	90.0	18.0
3. Records/documentation	10.0	92.0	9.2
4. Equipment maintenance	20.0	95.0	19.0
5. Bacteriological measurements	NA	NA	NA
6. Public relations	20.0	88.0	17.6
7. Area maintenance	10.0	75.0	7.5
Totals	100.0		88.3

Figure 5-5. Quality Inspection Instructions and Report: Physical Medicine Department

Block 5: Enter the period number and period dates from the Quality/Productivity Data Input Record: for example, 6/87, 11/17–12/14/86.

Block 6: The individual who conducts the quality inspections for this period should enter his or her name in this block.

Block 7: Enter the dates when the inspections were conducted: up to 8 different dates can be entered.

The dates selected for the performance of inspections should be representative of the reporting period, reference block 5,

Week 1—Sunday/Monday
Week 2—Tuesday/Wednesday
Week 3—Thursday/Friday
Week 3—Saturday/Sunday

for example:

2/4	2/12	2/15	2/20
2/25	2/28	3/1	3/3

Block 9: The "Class number" is used to determine the number of observations to be made in regard to each question during each 4-week period:

Class I (Critical):
A minimum of 5 observations MUST be made.

Classes 2 and 3 (Major and Minor): A minimum of 5 observations SHOULD be made.

Block 11: Enter the results of each observation for the **corresponding period** in the applicable column. The entries should be in tally form:

Yes	No	Total
|||	||	⫟⫟

After all of the observations have been completed for the reporting period, the tally should be totaled and the resulting totals entered and circled in each column:

Yes	No	Total
|||③	||②	⑤

After all of the observations have been completed for the period, the totals should be entered in the applicable area:

1. **Procedural Totals:**

Yes	No	Total
20	18	38

These entries should be entered into Section A of the Quality/Productivity Data Input Record.

Filing Procedures

The completed Quality Inspection Instructions and Report should be on file in your cost center or department for 12 months. After 12 months it can be discarded.

The Management Services Department will conduct periodic audits regarding these reports to verify the data entered on the Quality/Productivity Data Input Record.

Continued on next page

Figure 5-5. Continued

1. Cost Center—description Physical Medicine	Date
2. Approved by Cost Center/Dept. Manager	Date
3. Approved by Management Services Department	Date
4. Approved by Subdiv./Div. Head	Date

Inspection Data

5. Period no.

6. Inspected by

7. Dates of inspections _____

8. Quality Characteristic	9. Class No.	10. Source Code	11. Observations Yes No Total	11. Observations Yes No Total	11. Observations Yes No Total	11. Observations Yes No Total
Procedural						
1. Are inpatient referrals responded to within 24 calendar hours of being written, excluding weekends?	2					
2. Are physicians notified in writing of treatment plan and patient progress via daily progress notes?	1					
3. Is a complete initial evaluation performed and documented within the first 2 treatment sessions?	2					
1. Procedural Totals						
Service						
1. Are all rehabilitation patients receiving 2 hours of physical therapy and 1 hour of occupational therapy daily, excluding weekends?	2					

8. Quality Characteristic	9. Class No.	10. Source Code	11. Observations Yes No Total	11. Observations Yes No Total	11. Observations Yes No Total	11. Observations Yes No Total
2. Are inpatient no-shows due to scheduling conflicts less than 35% of transport schedule?	2					
2. **Service Totals:**						
3. **Records**						
1. Are billing sheets turned in and charges entered on a daily basis?	2					
2. Are patient treatment goals documented during initial evaluation?	2					
3. Is patient education documented?						
3. **Records Totals:**						
4. **Public Relations**						
1. Is the telephone answered courteously?	2					
2. Do all staff exhibit a sensitive, caring, and helpful attitude in dealing with patients, visitors, and hospital personnel?	2					
3. Do all staff exhibit effective communication skills when dealing with problems or complaints?	2					
4. **Public Relations Totals:**						
5. **Physical Environment**						
1. Are patient care areas neat and orderly?	3					
2. Are floors clean and dry?	2					
5. **Physical Environment Totals:**						

observation. For example, a major medical center made the following investment in a quality-management program during a recent fiscal year:

Type of Investment	Annual Amount
Cost center specific	$ 150,000
Malpractice insurance	3,700,000
Other (committees, and so forth)	200,000
Total	$4,050,000
Quality Investment as a % of Net Revenue:	2.3%

By itself, the 2.3 percent investment in quality at this medical center
is not an interesting statistic. It becomes interesting when it is compared
with the average for the manufacturing industry, which invests 20 percent
of its net revenue in quality. [The data for the manufacturing industry are
taken from a recent article by Ryan (1987).] The manufacturing industry,
on average, expended almost nine times as much as this medical center did
on a quality-management program. Experience in the manufacturing industry indicates that a larger investment is required at the start of such a program. The experience further indicates that quality-management costs, if
managed correctly, should decrease over time in response to an aggressive
quality-management program. On the basis of the author's experience in
both manufacturing and health care, this example clearly shows that this
medical center has not yet begun to invest enough in a total quality-
management program.

Within the manufacturing industry, the cost of quality management typically includes the following:

- *Appraisal costs,* including the inspection and testing of incoming
  materials, inspection and testing within the manufacturing processes,
  final product testing, and other testing procedures
- *Prevention costs,* including the development of product quality standards, maintenance of quality inspection instructions, quality engineering costs, and so on
- *Failure costs,* including scrap, rework, and repair of products which
  do not meet quality standards; lost sales associated with not meeting
  the customer's expectations in the market; product liability costs,
  including liability insurance; and so on

The cost data taken from the medical center do not include all of the costs
associated with the manufacturing industry. These other costs exist, but the
current information systems within health care organizations do not support the routine recording and reporting of these cost data. If these other
cost data were available, the total cost of quality management for the

medical center would still be significantly lower than the average for a manufacturing business.

Department-Level Commitment

Ideally, a facilitywide quality-management program requires a supporter at the senior executive level. This supporter must possess the requisite authority and power to be able to champion the program. If an executive supporter does not exist, department managers can still develop and implement quality-management programs within their own departments. In many health care facilities, department heads are allowed enough management flexibility to accomplish this assignment. As the earlier case on the radiology charting process illustrated, these programs usually do not require a significant capital investment or an extensive investment in labor, because in many applications the required inspection data already exist. The analysis of these data is the only additional activity usually required by personnel already employed by the department. If additional staff resources need to be directed in support of the quality-management program, the return on this investment will more than justify the expenditure.

Other Considerations

When planning for the implementation of a quality-management program, whether facilitywide or department focused, the executive or lower-level manager needs to assess how fast the program can be implemented, in other words, the rate of implementation. Typically, program implementation can proceed at a much faster rate in community or teaching-affiliated facilities than in academic medical centers. Many factors account for this difference, but the specifics are beyond the scope of this chapter. Differences in these rates are largely a function of management capability more than any other factor. If a manager is committed to the program, almost anything is possible. As with any type of management program, the employees, whether senior managers or rank-and-file technicians, will quickly assess their supervisor's level of commitment to the program. All employees exhibit a fairly universal trait: They pay attention to what the boss pays attention to. The message for the manager, whether the chief executive officer or the chief technician, is the same: If you want the program to be successful, pay attention to it.

Another good strategy, which is not unique to quality-management programs, is to have employees participate in the development of the program material. Participation builds commitment. Participation does not work well in every situation, but as a rule of thumb, it should always be considered.

Steps in the Planning and Implementation Process

As with any new program development assignment, planning the approach to implementing a quality-management program is often overlooked in order to get going on the assignment itself. The urge to get going as soon as possible should be resisted until a plan to complete the required work has been developed and reviewed with all individuals who will have a stake in the outcome. In summary, the steps within the following four phases should be determined in detail at the start of the assignment:

1. Organize and manage the assignment.
2. Develop the quality-management program.
3. Implement the program.
4. Maintain the program so that it is up-to-date.

One of the items developed during phase 1 is the work plan. Work plans typically detail the following information:

- The work tasks to be completed
- The responsibility(ies) for the completion of each task (one person is ultimately responsible for the completion of a task even when the responsibility is shared with more than one person)
- The estimated start-up and completion date for each task

In some cases, work plans should also detail the output that is produced when the task is completed. In consulting jargon, output is known as *the deliverable*. A sample work plan for the development and implementation of a quality reporting program for a department or a function within a department is table 5-3. In this example, an output was not detailed for each task. The hypothetical schedule included in this example can be used as a general guideline for this type of assignment. Of course, the schedule and tasks can be modified to suit individual circumstances.

The work plan illustrated in table 5-3 would need to be modified if the assignment were to address the development and implementation of a quality-management program at a facilitywide level. A work plan for a facilitywide program is provided in figure 5-6. As shown, this example does not detail the individual tasks within each subphase, and the scope of this assignment included the concurrent development of a facilitywide productivity program. This program emphasized the training of all of the participants: department heads, middle managers, and senior executives. As with any management program, the training and development needs of the participants require careful evaluation during the initial planning phase of the assignment. As stated earlier, most health care managers have not received any formal or informal (on-the-job) training on quality or productivity measurement techniques. This statement also applies to most senior health care executives. In many management training programs, the comment heard all too often is, "Boy, my boss should attend this program. If this program is so important, why isn't he here?"

Table 5-3. Sample Work Plan for the Development of a Departmental Quality Program

Task	Responsibility	Estimated Start Date	Estimated Completion Date
#1. Identify participants; obtain commitment to participate	Department head	3/7	3/11
#2. Complete initial research on the assignment	Department head	3/7	3/18
#3. Schedule and conduct the first participant team meeting; review the scope and *objectives* of the assignment, including *report design requirements;* confirm responsibilities for specific tasks	Department head	3/14	3/25
#4. Document the current process: prepare a flow diagram; collect all related forms, etc.; review with participants as required	Department head	3/28	4/8
#5. Identify inspection characteristics and inspection points on the flow diagram; identify data sources	Department head, participants	4/4	4/15
#6. Develop quality inspection instructions: determine sampling plans; revise related forms/reports if necessary to incorporate required data	Department head, participants	4/18	4/29
#7. Schedule and conduct the second participant team meeting; review the output from tasks 4, 5, and 6; confirm same	Department head, participants	5/2	5/6
#8. Conduct a staff meeting, if necessary, or meet individually with employees whose duties will change; review new/revised procedures as required	Department head, staff	5/9	5/13
#9. Implement the Quality Inspection and Results Reporting Program; monitor the program on a daily basis	Department head, participants	5/16	7/1
#10. Compile and review results to date; schedule and conduct the third participant team meeting; review the results; identify changes, if any; incorporate changes	Department head, participants	7/4	7/15
#11. Incorporate status reports on the program into regularly scheduled staff meetings	Department head	7/18	Ongoing

One other item that is often overlooked by the senior executive group within a health care facility is program maintenance. Quality-management programs require ongoing maintenance, whether they are specific to an individual department or are facilitywide. *Maintenance,* when used in this context, is defined as the allocation of staff resources either within the department or on a central, facilitywide level. In many cases, management engineers can assist a department manager during the development of a departmental

Figure 5-6.   Facilitywide Work Plan for the Development and Implementation of a Quality/Productivity Management Program

Phase 1: Organize and Manage the Assignment
Subphase 1.1. Develop and obtain approval of a program proposal
Subphase 1.2. Manage the assignment

Phase 2: Procure Work Measurement Standards Data System and Quality/Productivity Reporting System Software
Subphase 2.1. Develop and release a request for proposal
Subphase 2.2. Evaluate and select a vendor
Subphase 2.3. Execute and manage a contract
Subphase 2.4. Receive and install the data system and software

Phase 3: Develop and Conduct Five Workshops
Subphase 3.1. Develop support materials and calendar schedule for each workshop
Subphase 3.2. Conduct Workshop #1: Introduction and Quality
Subphase 3.3. Conduct Workshop #2: Productivity Management
Subphase 3.4. Conduct Workshop #3: Data Input and Reports
Subphase 3.5. Conduct Workshop #4: Review of Workshops 1, 2, and 3
Subphase 3.6. Conduct work sampling studies in three departments
Subphase 3.7. Conduct Workshop #5: Performance Analysis and Review Report

Phase 4: Activate the Quality/Productivity Reporting System
Subphase 4.1. Develop the data input and standards maintenance system
Subphase 4.2. Implement the productivity data input system
Subphase 4.3. Implement the quality inspection program and data input system
Subphase 4.4. Distribute productivity reports
Subphase 4.5. Distribute quality reports

Phase 5: Implement a Revised Position Control System
Subphase 5.1. Document current system
Subphase 5.2. Design Revised System
Subphase 5.3. Implement Revised System

program or provide centrally based consulting services during the development of a facilitywide program. In this capacity, the management engineer is providing quality engineering services in support of the program. The use of engineers in this capacity is not new. Quality engineering was established as a profession during World War II. Since that time, the profession has grown to employ approximately 25,000 professionals on a national level in all types of industries, including service delivery industries.

Quality engineers usually provide the following services:

- Development and ongoing maintenance of quality inspection instructions and reports

- Completion of special statistical studies, including the determination of statistically valid sample sizes and process capability studies
- Guidance of managers in the interpretation of quality-measurement results and the completion of special investigations into the cause of quality deficiencies

The amount of management/quality engineering resources required to support a quality-management program depends upon the scope of the pro- gram as measured by the number of departments, functions, or processes included in the program, as well as the extent of the use of various quality data analysis techniques. As an approximate rule of thumb, the following allocation is suggested: 10.0 work hours per month per department or func- tion or process program maintained. For example, the following calcula- tion can be carried out for 10 department-level programs:

10 programs × 10 hours per program per month × 12 months per year =

1,200 work hours per year × 1.12 benefit time adjustment =

1,344 paid hours per year/2,080 paid hours per year per FTE =

0.6 FTE

(The benefit time adjustment is for sick, vacation, and holiday time.) The above maintenance allocation does not reflect the time spent on conduct- ing quality inspections at the department, function, or process level. This estimate only reflects the time spent by the quality engineer in providing ongoing technical support services.

Upon review, an allocation of a 0.6 full-time equivalent (FTE) may seem insignificant; however, when it is viewed as a percentage of the total resources available in the typical management engineering department, it is not insig- nificant. If it is assumed that the typical department has a professional staff- ing complement of 4.0 FTEs, this allocation represents 16 percent of the total staffing complement. This allocation does not include any support that may have been provided by the management engineering staff during the original development of the quality-management program. The need to allo- cate engineering resources in an ongoing manner may not be well received nor understood by senior management.

Evaluation of Results and Outcomes

During the development of the quality-management program, considera- tion must be given to the identification of information that can support the quality performance analysis and decision-making process. In this con- text, this analysis and decision-making process is managerial in nature rather than rank and file oriented. After a program has been in operation for some time, say one to two years for a facilitywide program or three to six months for a department- or process-focused program, the process can be extended to the rank-and-file employee level. If an individual manager thinks that employees can be brought into the analysis and decision-making process sooner, he or she should do so.

Required Information

When designing quality inspection programs, the manager must initially focus on the types of information that will be required to support the evaluation of performance and the corresponding improvement of performance when indicated. All too often, a manager will jump into the design of the data collection forms without first considering the objectives of the program. If this occurs, the manager does not realize that he or she has overlooked critical data elements until the first or second set of performance reports has been generated. The incorporation of these additional data elements, at best, is difficult and possibly not feasible (for example, in the case of an automated system) at this stage in the development of the program. The need to consider the output from the inspection program at the beginning of the development process cannot be overemphasized.

The typical quality-management reporting system should provide the following types of information:

- Trend data (that is, time-series data both in the form of a statistical table and as a graph). If the reports are produced by some form of an automated system (spreadsheet application software or custom-designed software), the reports should include the calculated least-squares regression slope. Figure 5-7 illustrates the use of the slope statistic.
- Variance data (that is, the comparison of actual to the expected standard or goal).
- Cause data (that is, data that may indicate why the process is not conforming to the required expectations). In some cases, cause data may not be included in the routine reports but would only be available as the result of a special quality investigation.
- Cost data (that is, quality cost data as described earlier in this chapter). These types of data may not be included in the initial reporting system but may be incorporated at a later date.

[For further information on these types of data, see Berger and Hart (1986), Hansen (1963), and Simmons (1972).]

A cost-center-level report developed by the medical center discussed earlier in this chapter is presented in figure 5-7. As shown, this report represents the application of a quality program at the department level using data compiled on the department's Quality Inspection Instructions and

Figure 5-7. Cost Center Quality Report

Quality Detailed Report
Period: 8/24/87 to 3/6/88
Division: 100002
Subdivision: 400021
Department: 500211—Rehabilitation
Cost Center: 1267741—Physical Medicine

Quality Characteristics	Relative Value (1)	Observed Score (2)	Current Quality Index 2/8 to 3/6/88 (1 × 2)
Procedural	30.0%	93.3	28.0%
Service	20.0%	100.0	20.0%
Records	20.0%	86.6	17.3%
Equipment	.0%	.0	.0%
Bacteriological measurements	.0%	.0	.0%
Public relations	12.5%	100.0	12.5%
Physical environment	17.5%	100.0	17.5%
Total quality index			95.3%
Moving average quality index for 13 periods			79.2%
Quality goal range			95.0%–100.0%

	Quality Indices for Last 6 Periods						
Quality Characteristics	8/24 to 9/20/87	9/21 to 10/18	10/19 to 11/15	11/16 to 12/13	12/14 to 1/10	1/11 to 2/7/88	Index Slope
Procedural	26.0%	22.0%	22.0%	22.0%	26.0%	26.0%	.64
Service	20.0%	20.0%	20.0%	20.0%	20.0%	20.0%	.00
Records	16.0%	16.0%	18.7%	18.7%	17.3%	17.3%	.19
Equipment	.0%	.0%	.0%	.0%	2.5%	.0%	.09
Bacteriological measurements	.0%	.0%	.0%	.0%	2.5%	.0%	.09
Public relations	9.3%	8.7%	10.0%	8.7%	10.0%	11.7%	.55
Physical environment	15.0%	15.0%	13.5%	15.0%	15.0%	17.5%	.50
Totals	86.3%	81.7%	84.2%	84.4%	93.3%	92.5%	2.06

Report (see figure 5-5). This report is produced on a personal computer using custom software supplied by an outside vendor. The quality index for each four-week reporting period is also displayed on a graphic report (figure 5-8). In addition to generating reports at the cost center level, this reporting software can generate reports at department (two or more cost centers), subdivision (two or more departments), division, and facility levels.

When reviewing the sample report presented in figure 5-7, note that the report presented in figure 5-1 (the Process Quality Control Record) also represents an effective report design. Although this report is limited in scope, it can be manually maintained, or it can be automated as a spreadsheet application using one of the popular, personal computer-based, commercial software packages. The report design presented in figure 5-7 for the physical

Figure 5-8. Cost Center Quality Graph

(Asterisk indicates that quality inspections were not performed)

Cost Center Report   Periods: 3/9/87–3/6/88

Division: 100002   Department: 500211–Rehabilitation   Cost Center: 1267741–Physical Medicine

QUALITY REPORT   QUALITY INDEX   Run Date: 3/25/88
Physical Medicine   Periods 4/5/87 to 3/6/88

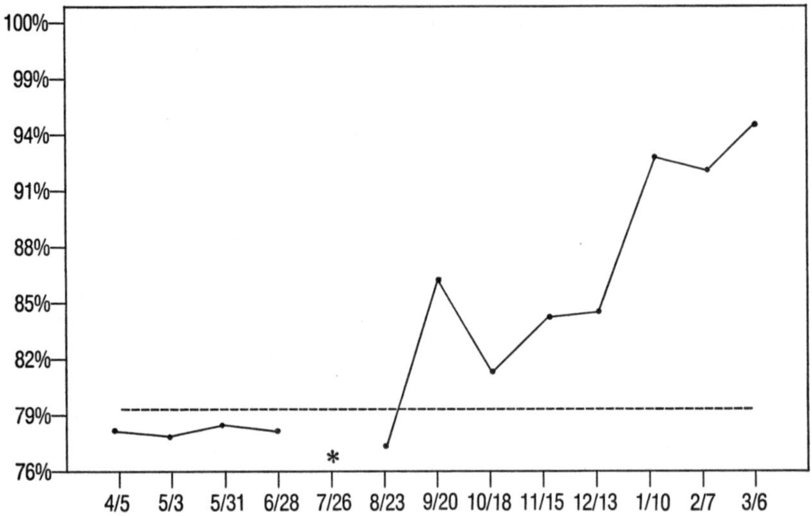

Goal Range 95.0%–100.0%   ———— Quality Index   ------- Average

medicine cost center in the Rehabilitation Department does not include quality cost data, nor does it include cause data (data that would help pinpoint
the cause of poor quality). This is pointed out to emphasize that many different alternatives are available for the design of quality performance reports.
There is no single best solution.

Process Capability Analysis

In the earlier discussion on the types of data that should be included in
the design of a quality reporting system, it was suggested that the reports
include variance data. The use of variance data appears to be an easy concept similar to the use of variance data in revenue- and expense-reporting systems. The use of quality-variance data in health care requires that some type
of a standard or goal needs to be determined or selected before any variances to actual data can be considered. A health care manager may ask where
these standards come from. Are they available from some outside regional,
state, or national organization? The answers to these questions are yes and no.

In every application of a quality-management program, a manager needs to determine what constitutes acceptable performance: acceptable to the patient (the customer) and acceptable to the industry as well. In most situations, no known standards of acceptable performance exist in the health care industry. When used in this context, the standards promulgated by the Joint Commission on the Accreditation of Healthcare Organizations (JCAHO) are excluded because in almost all cases, the JCAHO standards are structural in nature, not outcome or process performance standards for a specific health care facility.

To respond to this apparent problem, it is beneficial to review the experience in other industries. The experience in other industries was similar when the quality engineering profession first started during World War II. Since that time, process capability analysis has received widespread use. According to Hansen (1963, p. 92), the purpose of a process capability analysis is to determine the "natural variation" of a process when the effects of all extraneous factors not contributing to the process have been minimized. Process capability may be defined as the "minimum spread of a specific quality characteristic which will statistically include 99.7 percent of the measurements from a given process," in other words, six standard deviations.

The results of a process capability analysis using the earlier example for the Radiology Report Charting process are presented in figure 5-9. As

Figure 5-9.   Process Capability Analysis: Radiology Report Charting Process

Examinations performed on Mon., Tue., Wed., or Thu.

Statistic: Elapsed hours from the time when the order is written by the physician to the time the result report is charted in the medical record.

Observation	Frequency of Occurrence	
52	5	
51	15	
50	15	
49	23	
48	12	
47	10	
46	3	
45	0	Mean = $\bar{X}$ = 48
44	0	
43	9	Standard Deviation (SD) = 3.09
42	5	
41	0	Process Capability = 6 × SD = 18.54
40	2	
39	0	
38	1	
	100	

discussed earlier, the chairman of the Radiology Department had stated that the standard for the charting of the reports in the medical chart was 24 hours. As admitted by this chairman, no one had ever attempted to determine what the process was capable of achieving. As shown in figure 5-9, the original charting process was not capable of achieving this given standard: The average time was 48 hours, with a process capability from 38.7 to 57.3 hours (48 ± 3 standard deviations). This capability study of the charting process used the results compiled from the initial study before the implementation of the process quality reporting program.

If after a process capability analysis has been completed, it is determined that the results (that is, the capability) of a process or department are not acceptable to the customers or the manager or both, the manager should review the process in more detail. The purpose of the detailed review is to determine where changes can be made in the process or department that will result in improved performance. Materials, systems, procedures, personnel, personnel work schedules, and so on should be evaluated, adjusted if indicated, and monitored after any changes to confirm that the process capability has indeed improved. If the capability has not improved, the change analysis cycle should be repeated or the expectations of the customer, the manager, or both should be adjusted if feasible.

Pareto's Law

Another analytical tool that can be used with great success in completing the detailed review is Pareto's law, which is also commonly referred to as ABC analysis. This law basically states that 20 percent of the quality characteristics will account for 80 percent of the quality problems, for example:

- 20 percent of the organization's surgeons will account for 80 percent of the operative case delays.
- 20 percent of the organization's personnel will account for 80 percent of the quality problems.
- 20 percent of the organization's stock items will account for 80 percent of the usage volume.
- 20 percent of the organization's physicians will account for 80 percent of the inpatient cases with average length of stays exceeding the regional average for the same diagnosis-related group (DRG).

Using Pareto's law will help a manager determine how to allocate his or her time in an effort to eliminate or minimize quality problems or deficiencies so that the manager will receive the best return on the time investment. Table 5-4 illustrates how Pareto's law was applied during a detailed review within the Utilization Management Department, which had developed a quality inspection program. (The design used was similar to the one illustrated for the Physical Medicine Department in figure 5-5.) Two (20 percent) of the quality inspection characteristics accounted for 70 percent of

Table 5-4. Application of Pareto's Law: Utilization Management Department

Question	Characteristic Description	Number of "No"s	Cumulative Number of "No"s	Percent of "No"s of Total
#3	Are all third-party payer admissions called in to the payer within an acceptable period after admission (24–72 hours)?	8	8	40.0% "8/20" × 100
#9	Are responses to state questions communicated within the prescribed time of 30 days? (Source: Log)	6	14 "8 + 6"	70.0% "14/20" × 100
#4	Are all cases reviewed prior to expiration of the previous extension? (Source: SMS Continued Stay Review Worksheet)	3	17 "14 + 3"	85.0%
#10	Is the billing office notified of any problems regarding third-party payment? (Source: Certification form or SMS Continued Stay Review Worksheet)	2	19	95.0%
#8	Are all cases being reviewed for appropriate level of care (LDC)? (Source: SMS Continued Stay Review Worksheet)	1	20	100.0%

Results: Two of your characteristics (#3 and #9) account for 70% of your problems.

the quality deficiencies as measured by this department's quality-management program. A detailed approach for the application of Pareto's law is provided in appendix B. (The example in appendix B is also for the Utilization Management Department using the data presented in table 5-4.)

Conclusion

When planning for the development of a quality program, health care managers need to realize that quality can be measured and that it must be measured and managed just like any other performance characteristic. The material presented in this chapter should be sufficient to initiate a quality-management program. If additional assistance is required, managers can consult the reference list and the management engineering/systems department of their organization. If managers have a strong interest in the field of quality management, they should consider becoming a member of the Health Care Committee, Administrative Applications Division, of the American Society for Quality Control (310 West Wisconsin Avenue, Milwaukee, WI 53203).

When evaluating the relationship between quality and productivity, health care managers need to realize that these are not mutually exclusive performance characteristics and that an improvement in productivity will not automatically result in a reduction in quality. If managed correctly, both of these characteristics can be improved at the same time.

The other thing to remember is that more is not necessarily always better than less, as Dorothy Rice points out in a recent article in *Hospitals* magazine (1988). The vast expenditures for medical care in this country, she says, are neither providing universal access nor the higher health status that many other developed countries enjoy for a proportionately smaller expenditure. She supports her position by presenting some interesting statistics.

A recent study of health care spending in the Organization for Economic Cooperation and Development (OECD) countries shows that the average per capita health care expenditure in 1985 for 22 developed countries was $848 in U.S. dollars, and the range went from $252 in Greece to $1,776 in the United States. Rice goes on to state that the real bottom line is whether our investment in health care provides improved health. If so, we may be getting value for our money. On the other hand, if the health status of our nation is below that of other nations that spend comparatively less, we might conclude that our medical care dollars are being spent inappropriately and that there might be considerable waste in the system.

One traditional health outcome indicator considered a surrogate for general health status is infant mortality, in which the United States ranks 15th among the 22 nations. Americans spend 2.2 times as much per capita for health care as the average for the other 21 countries. Yet our infant mortality rates are as much as 1.7 times higher, according to Rice.

Life expectancy at birth shows similar patterns. The United States ranks 12th among the nations for men and 9th for women. Japan has the longest life expectancy, and its per capita expenditure for health is less than half of ours. Such statistics are worth pondering as health care managers pursue the establishment of their own quality-management programs.

References

Berger, R., and Hart, T. *Statistical Process Control—A Guide for Implementation.* New York City: Marcel Dekker, ASQC Quality Press, 1986.

Berry, L., Zeithaml, V., and Parasuraman, A. Quality counts in services, too. *Business Horizons* 28(3):44–52, May–June 1985.

Gitlow, H. S., and Gitlow, G. J. *The Deming Guide to Quality and Competitive Position.* Englewood Cliffs, NJ: Prentice-Hall, 1987.

Hansen, B. *Quality Control: Theory and Applications.* Englewood Cliffs, NJ: Prentice-Hall, 1963.

King, C. A framework for a service quality assurance system. *Quality Progress,* Sept. 1987, pp. 27–32.

Miller, M. C., III, and Knapp, R. G. *Evaluating Quality of Care—Analytic Procedures—Monitoring Techniques.* Germantown, MD: Aspen Systems Corp., 1979.

Rice, D. Do we get full value for our health dollar? *Hospitals* 62(6):18, Mar. 20, 1988.

Ryan, J. 1987 ASQC/Gallup survey. *Quality Progress,* Dec. 1987, pp. 13–17.

Simmons, D. *Medical and Hospital Control Systems—The Critical Difference.* Boston, MA: Little, Brown and Co., 1972.

Appendix A. Sample Size Selection Instructions

Standard Instructions

The *Department Head* or authorized designee will review page 1 of the Quality Inspection Instructions and Report (QII&R) (figure 5-5). This person should review the "Class No." column (Block 9) to determine the class number assignment for each question.

If the class number assignment is 1, a *minimum* of 5 observations MUST be made during the 4-week inspection period.

If the class number assignment is 2 or 3, a *minimum* of 5 observations SHOULD be made during the 4-week inspection period.

Special Instructions

If in the judgment and experience of the *Department Head,* a sample size greater than 5 observations is appropriate, the *Department Head* or authorized designee will then:

1. Review the "Class No." column on the QII&R to determine the class number assignment for each question.
2. If the class number assignment is 1, determine the average inspection unit population volume for each question for a 4-week reporting period. NOTE: Step 1 can also be applied to Class 2, *Major,* and Class 3, *Minor,* questions.
3. Review table A-1 and select the applicable sample size for each question reviewed in step 1.
4. Select the number of units, occurrences, and so forth, in accordance with the selected sample size, in a *random* manner representative of the activity being inspected over the 4-week period.

Example 1: Utilization Management

1. Procedural:

Question 3.   Are all third-party payer admissions called in to the payer within an acceptable period after admission?

Average Inspection Unit Population:
            1,300 third-party payer admissions processed in a 4-week period

Sample Size: 125 from line 10 on table A-1 to be inspected in each 4-week period

---

Example 2: Physical Medicine

1. Procedural:

Question 2.   Are physicians notified in writing of treatment plan and patient progress via daily progress notes?

Average Inspection Unit Population:
            2,000 patient visits to Physical Medicine in a 4-week period

Sample Size: 125 from line 10 on table A-1 to be inspected in each 4-week period

---

Example 3: Endoscopy

2. Service:

Question 1. Do patients arrive in Endoscopy properly prepared for the procedure?

Average Inspection Unit Population:
100 patient visits to Endoscopy requiring a prep in a 4-week period

Sample size: 20 from line 6 on table A-1 to be inspected in each 4-week period

---

Example 4: Purchasing

7. Physical Environment:

Question 1. Are floors maintained in a clean and safe condition?
NOTE: Environmental Services dry mops the floors each workday.

Average Inspection Unit Population:
20 dry-mop occurrences in a 4-week period (5 workdays per week × 4 weeks)

Sample size: 5 from line 3 on table A-1 to be inspected in each 4-week period

---

Table A-1. Sample Size Selection Table

Inspection Unit Population Volume per 4-Week Period		Sample Size
1.	2 to 8	2
2.	9 to 15	3
3.	16 to 25	5
4.	26 to 50	8
5.	51 to 90	13
6.	91 to 150	20
7.	151 to 280	32
8.	281 to 500	50
9.	501 to 1,200	80
10.	1,201 to 3,200	125
11.	3,201 to 10,000	200
12.	10,001 to 35,000	315

Source: Sampling Procedures and Tables for Inspection by Attributes, U.S. Government Printing Office, publication no. MIL-STD-105D.

Appendix B. Application of Pareto's Law — A Case Example

Step #1: Rank the results of your quality inspections.

(1) Review the Quality Inspection Instructions and Report (QII&R) (figure 5-5) for your cost center for the past three reporting periods, that is, the most recent 12-week period.

(2) Compile the number of "No" responses for *class 1* quality characteristics (questions) for *one* of the seven standard inspection categories. Select the category based upon which characteristic has the largest *negative* index slope and the quality score as it compares to the relative index.

(3) Rank order the resulting *class 1* quality characteristics from the highest number of "No"s to the lowest.

(4) Calculate the cumulative *number* of "No"s by characteristic.

(5) Calculate the cumulative *percent* of "No"s by characteristic.

Example: Utilization Management — QII&R

Period:	09/87–11/87 (2/9/87–5/3/87)
Category:	1–Procedural
Class:	1–Critical

Question Number	Characteristic Description	Number of "No"s	Cumulative Number of "No"s	Cumulative Percent of Total
#3	Are all third-party payer admissions called in to the payer within an acceptable period after admission (24–72 hours)?	8	8	40.0% "8/20" × 100
#9	Are responses to state questions communicated within the prescribed time of 30 days? (Source: Log)	6	14 "8 + 6"	70.0% "14/20" × 100
#4	Are all cases reviewed prior to expiration of the previous extension? (Source: SMS Continued Stay Review Worksheet)	3	17 "14 + 3"	85.0%
#10	Is the billing office notified of any problems regarding third-party payment? (Source: Certification form or SMS Continued Stay Review Worksheet)	2	19	95.0%
#8	Are all cases being reviewed for appropriate level of care (LDC)? (Source: SMS Continued Stay Review Worksheet)	1	20	100.0%

Results: Two of your characteristics (#3 and #9) account for 70% of your

Step #2: Examine the questions and cost center conditions to determine (best guess) where the problem lies.

Problem	Solution
The system/procedure?	Change them.
The materials?	Change them.
The equipment?	Change/repair it.
The employee/patient?	Train/educate them.

Step #3: Develop a quality improvement action plan.

(1) Determine (guess at) the *cause* of the quality problem.

(2) Prepare an *outline* describing how you intend to eliminate/minimize the "cause."
   — Solicit help from your employees. Remember, they work with the situation all of the time. They may have some very good answers on how to solve the problem once they are made aware of the problem.

(3) Review the outline with your immediate supervisor and finalize your quality improvement action plan. Include the following within the quality improvement action plan:
   — *Interface requirements* if they exist with other departments/cost centers.
   — An estimated *schedule* for the execution of the "Action Plan."

Example: Utilization Management — Quality Improvement Action Plan

Problem — Characteristic #3: Are all third-party payer admissions called in to the payer within an acceptable period after admission (24–72 hours)?

(1) Determine (guess at) the cause: There is an apparent delay in determining the payer in a timely manner.
   Why?
   — Information is not correct on the admission form.
   — Employees are not aware of the need to call within the time frame.
   — The results of a one-week data collection program indicate that the employees in the Admissions Office are incorrectly recording the payer.
   — Six problems were reported out of 20 patients admitted that week.

(2) Prepare an outline: There is a need to develop and/or conduct an inservice training program for the employees in the Admissions Office.

(3) Finalize the Quality Improvement Action Plan.

   (a) Involve departments/individuals
      — Business Office Manager
      — Director, Hospital Admissions
      — Employees of Hospital Admissions Department
      — Manager, Training and Development

(b) Estimated Completion Schedule
    —Develop or improve the training program in conjunction with the training and development function. (For example, Director, Hospital Admissions: 0–2 weeks.)
    —Conduct training sessions for employees from all shifts. (For example, Manager, Training and Development: 2–3 weeks.)

Step #4: Implement the action plan and *monitor* the results via your quality inspection program.

(1) Were the "problems" eliminated/minimized?

(2) If *not, repeat* Steps 1–4

(3) Implement the action plan and *monitor* the results.
    —Plan implemented on schedule? Are the results acceptable?
    —If *not*, repeat the steps.

Chapter 6

Employment and Recruitment

Glenda M. Westbrook

Introduction

Just imagine for a moment that you have been named president of your organization. Here are a few of your problems:

- You operate a business that depends upon government contracts.
- You have no chance to make bids or negotiate prices.
- Your billings depend upon the availability of government funds.
- You will be paid a flat rate for services, no matter how extensive they are.
- If you make a profit, your payments will be reduced next year.
- You depend on a shrinking supply of professionals who are becoming increasingly disillusioned and who demand recognition and rewards consistent with their professional preparation and daily contribution to your customers.
- Social forces and public policy create increasing demands for your services and products while regulating the level of payment suppliers will receive.
- If you fail or falter in any step of the process of delivering your products and services, the likelihood of unreasoned, passionate, public outcry is great.
- You are responsible for human life in a disturbingly complex social environment that asks who should live, who should die, and who should decide and that expects your organization to discover and promulgate acceptable answers to these extraordinarily difficult questions.

How would you run this business? How would you position it to withstand the psychological dislocations these protean conditions suggest? How
would you manage the relentless clash of economic, social, and political
forces? How would you make your business plans coherent in the minds
of your various stakeholders, particularly to the employees who are the point
of contact with your customers and whose skills are in short supply and
high demand?

There are approximately 5,800 businesses operating in the United States
that, with few exceptions, fit a profile like the one just described. They are
America's hospitals. Their services, combined with those of other health
care providers, constitute 11 percent of the country's gross national product.
The preceding troubling description was adapted from a 1988 case study
formulated by the Center for Health Policy Research of the Oklahoma Medical Research Foundation (1988). The National Committee for Quality Health
Care has proposed a similar and even darker scenario in its report, *Critical
Condition—America's Healthcare in Jeopardy* (Rubin and others, 1988).

In such an environment, today's health care employees probably
experience frustration, anger, dismay, anxiety, and discouragement as part
of each workday. Paradoxically, it is also likely that they experience gratifi-
cation, excitement, success, fulfillment, and challenge.

Assessment, Selection, and the Productivity Challenge

Within this climate of ambiguity and turmoil, the health care manager faces
the most significant opportunities of recent history. As more and more people
inside and outside the industry contend with the cacophony, a rising need
for renewal and hope exists. Thoughtful, resourceful, steady, and perhaps
even obsessive attention from management has never been needed more.

Managers in health care organizations have become increasingly sophisticated in responding to many organizational demands. In fact, indications
are that managers seem to be quite good, and are getting better, at answering questions about why the work should be done, how it should be done,
how much it is worth to get it done, what sort of climate in which to do
the work should prevail, whether the right methods are used, and whether
the desired results are achieved. However, one fundamental question often
is overlooked or unspecified. It is the most basic of all questions any manager
must ask before any work can be accomplished: Who should do this work,
and how will we know that they can succeed?

A probing look at answers to this basic question can spur higher levels
of interest in the process of good employee selection. A secondary question
must then also be posed: Can our organizations depend on us to identify
talented, dedicated, spirited, attentive, and appropriate people to perform
the work of our enterprises? If a fully prepared, productive work force is
to be assured for the next decade, the health care manager must place an

overarching importance upon the assessment, selection, and retention of individuals who will make the most and best contributions. Without this strategic emphasis, the organization's success could be compromised. Robert and Joyce Hogan (1986, p. 1), both associated with the University of Tulsa, have said:

> The characteristics of successful organizations are reasonably well-known, and these characteristics can be summarized in one statement: Organizations are successful largely because good people work for them. Consequently, the quickest way to improve organizational performance is to improve the performance of people in them . . . through training or *selection.* (emphasis added)

In general, managers have access to far more knowledge in the area of assessment and selection than they are applying (Arvey and Campion, 1982). Further, organizations that have recognized the relevance of candidate assessment and selection to the success of the enterprise report dramatic results.

Florida Power Corporation, an electric utility in St. Petersburg, is one such company. Walt Thurn, manager of employee development, reports that before the establishment of a careful preemployment program, turnover in one critical position known as groundman was 48.3 percent. "Now, just five years later, with the preemployment program in full swing, turnover is a scant 4.5 percent," says Chris Lee, managing editor of *Training* (Feuer and Lee, 1988, pp. 30–31). Just as important, even with an increase in customers of 4.5 percent annually, "Sixteen percent fewer groundmen than in 1983 handle the increased work load . . . with a 65 percent decrease in the accident rate." Before the new selection and assessment program at Florida Power, a groundman required an average of 7.2 years to become a journeyman; now the promotion is earned in less than four years, on average.

Perhaps you believe that your organization's assessment and selection activities are energetic and prosperous. If so, this chapter may serve as positive reinforcement. However, you may believe that your organization's performance in this aspect of management is merely respectable or even less than respectable. If so, this exploration could provide the impetus for you to give higher priority than ever to the assessment and selection of employees.

In this chapter, I will address the economic impact enhanced assessment and selection potentially have. I will briefly discuss the importance of human resources planning and forecasting, especially during times of labor shortages. Further, I will explore the availability of some assessment and selection tools utilized by many successful companies, large and small. These tools are readily available or adaptable to health care organizations.

I will not discuss retention issues in detail. This subject is treated in other chapters in this book. Specifically, I refer the reader to chapters 1 and 8, which discuss corporate culture and recognition/reward, respectively. Also, I will not discuss the nursing shortage per se because it has been documented by others in numerous publications. However, all of the methods I discuss are applicable to the assessment and selection of nurses.

Economic Impact of Enhanced Assessment and Selection

Florida Power Corporation provides some of the most recent and compelling data on the economic benefits of careful employee selection. The corporation's lower turnover and accident rates, shorter training period, and greater productivity have saved the utility more than $1,200,000 since 1984, according to figures published in *Training* (Feuer and Lee, 1988), with a cost of less than $115,000 during the same period.

In my own hospital, during one year, we calculated that if we could reduce the number of new hires required because people left jobs owing to performance problems or dissatisfaction during the first year of employment, we could save as much as a quarter of a million dollars a year. We arrived at this projected savings through the creation of what we called a productivity effectiveness cost report. A sample of such a report is included as figure 6-1.

Of course, most large hospitals and institutions already have multiple mechanisms for collecting, analyzing, and distributing information regarding terminations and accessions. If so, these tools should receive new attention. However, rearranging data into a productivity effectiveness cost report can stimulate interest and curiosity, leading to problem identification and new objectives. Hence, developing a productivity effectiveness cost report could be beneficial.

Managers in small hospitals may have to invest a little time in collecting the required information. If you work in a small hospital that has someone assigned to personnel functions, be sure to check with that individual(s) regarding whether some of the information you need is already collected. Conversely, if you are a human resources professional in a small hospital, you will want to align yourself with several managers who are interested in collaborating on developing such a productivity effectiveness cost report.

To create a productivity effectiveness cost report for your institution or department, you will first need to gather some basic data. These data should be chosen from a period of time (a recent year or more) that will yield what you consider to be data useful for your own purposes. The basic data are:

- Salaries or estimated salaries of any persons who work full-time or part-time on recruitment, interviewing, and related activities (direct costs)
- Costs or estimated costs of all advertising (direct costs)

Figure 6-1. Sample Productivity Effectiveness Cost Report

1. Direct costs	$170,000	(Salaries of recruiters, receptionists; costs of advertising, travel, orientation, and so forth)
2. Indirect costs	$1,514,890	(Includes productivity effectiveness cost [PEC] computed below [$3,448 PEC × 430 hires = $1,482,640] plus cost of estimated interview time from managers [3 hours × $25 per hour × 430 new hires = $32,250])
3. Total costs	$1,684,890	
4. Total new hires	430	
5. Direct costs per hire	$395	($170,000÷430)
6. Indirect costs per hire	$3,523	($1,514,890÷430)
7. Total cost per new hire	$3,918	($1,684,890÷430)

Assumptions:
Average management hourly salary = $25
Average management interview time = 3 hours per hire
Average salary of new hires = $9 per hour = $360 per week
Percentages of effectiveness/productivity for first 24 weeks on job:
First　　8 weeks = 30% effective/productive
Second 8 weeks = 60%
Third　　8 weeks = 90%

Computation of Productivity Effectiveness Cost (PEC):
PEC = (No. of weeks) × (Average weekly rate of new hire) × (100% less the percentage of effective/productive performance for each of the first three 8-week periods):
First　　8 weeks: 8 weeks × $360 = $2,880 × .70 = $2,016
Second 8 weeks: 8 weeks × $360 = $2,880 × .40 =　1,152
Third　　8 weeks: 8 weeks × $360 = $2,880 × .10 = ___280
　　　　　　　　　　　　　　　　　PEC per hire　$3,448

- Costs or estimated costs of all travel related to recruitment and interviewing that the hospital pays for (direct costs)
- Salaries or estimated salaries and estimated time of all staff providing general hospital orientation programs (direct costs)
- Estimation of management interview time per hire (indirect costs)
- Estimated or average hourly management wage (indirect costs)
- Estimated or average hourly wage of new hires (indirect costs)
- Estimated number of weeks required for new hires to be 30/60/90 percent effective when compared with experienced and high-performing individuals in the same work unit

In the sample provided in figure 6-1, the number of weeks for each incremental improvement in effectiveness (or productivity) is eight weeks. However, it is conceivable that each hospital or unit/department therein will have a different amount of time during which a new hire is expected to be fully productive.

Once the productivity effectiveness costs are known, managers should analyze the terminations during a recent year to reveal those situations in which individuals left employment because of performance problems (which indicates a possible flaw in assessment and selection) or dissatisfaction with the job. The number of such terminations times the total cost per new hire (line 7 from the Productivity Effectiveness Cost Report) yields the potential savings if improved assessment and selection methods result in fewer terminations because of poor performance or job dissatisfaction.

Obviously, the more precise your information is, the more precise will be your baseline, against which you can measure the organization's success in lowering its employee turnover rate. In large organizations, the information will likely be much more accessible. However, even estimates can be a powerful tool to portray the economic opportunities in improved assessment and selection. As John Hendrickson (1987, p. 71) has said, " . . . The time has come . . . to re-focus on . . . the advantages of a more strategic assessment . . . it makes economic sense. A bad hiring decision costs thousands of dollars."

Human Resources Planning and Forecas⁺'ng in Troubled Times

Manzini and Gridley (1986, p. 250) provide much guidance regarding what we can do to close the apparent gaps between today's skills and talents and those needed to meet strategic plans and operational needs. According to them, "Changing technology, as well as changing markets, can produce unplanned and often unforeseeable demands for a different mix of skills than are being produced. . . . While some skills . . . are becoming outworn or obsolete, other skills and qualifications may be needed in greater supply." It would be difficult to find a better description of the dilemma felt by many health care managers and human resources professionals.

Shortages in labor supplies are typically a problem that must be addressed according to the characteristics of each situation. Depending on the organization, its position in the market, the size and scope of its activities, the availability of resources, and the rapidity of technological advances within its industry, one institution may be better positioned than another to cope with this issue. In general, however, as Manzini and Gridley point out, five major methods can be used to close gaps created by shortages. They are:

- *Turnover control programs,* which are "at the heart of any system that focuses on the internal availability of personnel and their development" (Manzini and Gridley, 1986, p. 251). Turnover control naturally follows from good data analysis. Such analysis can be sophisticated or simple, depending on the size of an organization. But the level of elaboration in the data analysis is less important than the rapidity with which managers move to control the avoidable departures of valuable personnel.

- *Accelerated development,* which normally includes "highly structured training or job experience along with increased responsibility" (Manzini and Gridley, 1986, p. 252) under expert tutelage. In large hospitals and systems, this method may be easier to institute because training and education departments can and should provide the consultation and expertise required. However, even in small hospitals, bright and productive people can be retained by allowing them to explore and try things they find challenging and by offering them opportunities to associate with other employees with whom they share expertise or desired skills/traits.

- *Long-range retraining and transfer,* which when increasing "technological advances displace workers, create job obsolescence . . . or result in large surpluses of human resources" (Manzini and Gridley, 1986, p. 252). One of the best examples of this concept in modern times is the massive and unprecedented changes resulting from the breakup of AT&T. Thousands of jobs were eliminated because of technological advances while thousands more that required new skills were created in geographically dispersed areas.

  Another modern example of this accelerated development is GenCorp Automotive, which is starting a new plant in Shelbyville, Indiana. The people hired to work there will all be salaried and will receive identical parking privileges, benefits, and gainsharing shares. The company seeks "people who will thrive in an environment of continual learning," says Ray Casper, director of human resources. "Further," he says, "the new plant won't have 48 different jobs. The entire work force will be able to do any job in the plant. People with this potential are the kind of people I'm going to select, train and develop" (Feuer and Lee, 1988, p. 24).

  Of course, except for hospitals that are part of health care systems, alliances, and networks, most hospitals believe that they must compete for human resources. This limits the appeal, scope, and results that long-range retraining and transfer might have on the national scale or for a company such as AT&T. Even so, thoughtful and successful managers will find ways to make a beginning by simply looking within their own departments for ways in which cross-training and transfers of skills and knowledge can be effected.

- *Leveraged technological skills,* which seek to spread the most technologically advanced personnel across the organization rather than concentrating them in a single unit or department. "If possible, the most technologically competent . . . should supervise groups of average or less advanced people. In firms with a limited supply of outstanding professionals, the utilization of these people as leaders can spread (or leverage) their skills and knowledge to a broader base" (Manzini and Gridley, 1986, p. 252). Within larger hospitals or systems, this seems to be a highly likely approach. Sometimes, institutions do this through the use of matrixing or product line management. Within smaller hospitals, this form of leveraged skill is probably already inherent in much of the day-to-day work just by the nature of a small organization. Being more conscious of this method, however, can ensure succession should the technologically competent person no longer be available.

• *External supply interventions*, which seek to attract new entrants into the labor pool through secondary and postsecondary education and training programs, community relations programs such as open houses, involvement in trade associations and business groups, and activities that promote positive attitudes about professions within an industry or toward the organization as a good place to work. Image enhancement campaigns may be seen as external supply interventions. Further, the manner in which a given organization presents itself in recruitment advertising can make a difference in the external supply of labor. Obviously, large hospitals or systems may have many resources through which to participate in these kinds of interventions. However, small hospitals, especially those in small towns, may be better positioned in the long run to develop an edge. Often, leaders at such hospitals are seen as stalwarts within their communities and hence are in a position to influence junior high and high school students. These students can be exposed to the inner workings of a hospital and encouraged to pursue health careers. One way to position students for your organization for the future is to seek gifts and endowments that could underwrite scholarships for students in return for service at your hospital upon completion of educational programs.

Assessment and Selection Techniques

I will discuss six specific assessment and selection techniques, each with distinct characteristics. Together they represent the range of possibilities available to managers today. Given the diversity of potential users, it must be left to the reader to discern which aspects of the techniques might be applicable to his or her situation. Additionally, these techniques are offered with the realization that a given organization might have or choose to have several valid assessment and selection procedures that, when combined, result in a systematic employment process.

    A study of these six approaches suggests that almost any organization, with a small investment of focused time, can enhance assessment and selection. Even if full-scale changes such as the Hogan Personnel Selection Series or the Expert Selection Program are not currently possible, some modified behavior among recruiters and interviewers could set the stage for future development. If nothing else, managers seeking to hire an employee can begin by asking themselves some questions before beginning the selection process. For example, what makes people successful in my department? What causes me to give up on some people? What didn't I like about the last applicants I talked with about an opening I had? What is the biggest problem I have with new hires? Your answers to these questions will help you focus your conversations with applicants and can serve as a framework for structuring an interview to help you find people who you think can succeed in your department, who possess the traits and skills you think are applicable to your open position, and who will be productive as quickly as possible.

Technique 1: Basic Testing

Simple skills tests are first among the tools available to enhance assessment and selection. In a recent survey of 245 companies conducted by the Bureau of National Affairs, Inc. (1988), 9 out of 10 employers reported that they administered such preemployment skills tests or examinations to applicants in at least one job category. For certain jobs within a hospital—no matter what the size of the hospital—the use of skills tests, such as for typing or word processing, and medical examinations seems clearly indicated and easy to accomplish.

After skills tests, medical examinations were the testing procedure used most often. For both skills tests and medical examinations, employers in the sample reported that applicants who fail these tests are disqualified from further consideration. Thirty-six percent of responding organizations had changed their testing practices in the three years before the survey, and the implementation of drug testing was the most commonly mentioned change.

Arvey (1979) and Arvey and Campion (1982) have notably provided literature searches and reviews on the subject of employment testing. I will not repeat these findings. It is sufficient to expect that assessment and selection tools and techniques must be valid and reliable and should not expose the organization to discrimination charges or other legal liabilities.

Many validated tests and assessment tools exist. Catalogs from suppliers can be obtained through your local library if you do not routinely receive them through the mail from your professional affiliations.

Technique 2: The Hogan Personnel Selection Series

The Hogan Personnel Selection Series (HPSS) is a series of empirically keyed measures of occupational performance derived from the Hogan Personality Inventory (Hogan, 1969). *The Hogan Personnel Selection Series Manual,* written by Joyce Hogan, Ph.D., and Robert Hogan, Ph.D. (1986, p. 1), gives a full description of the HPSS and the supportive research as well as sample reports. According to the Hogans, "Certain attitudes, values and motives are associated with competent performance in virtually any job. Three constellations of attitudes and values are particularly important and we call them Service Orientation, Reliability, and Stress Tolerance."

"Service Orientation characterizes employees who are attentive, pleasant, courteous and responsive to customer needs," say the Hogans. "Further, these employees are likable, popular and contribute to high morale." Reliability concerns "theft and organizational delinquency and refers to the attitudes, values and motives associated with maturity, conscientiousness and self-control as well as the ability to adapt to company policies. Reliability characterizes employees who are trustworthy and good organizational citizens" (Hogan and Hogan, 1986, p. 1).

"Persons characterized as having low stress tolerance are likely to become ill, to be involved in accidents, and to miss work because of medical considerations" (Hogan and Hogan, 1986, p. 1). For obvious reasons, high stress tolerance is a desirable trait in all employees, especially those working in health care.

The Hogans' research suggests that the kinds of people who perform well within various organizational roles are "people who are service oriented, reliable, and stress tolerant. Such people can be identified through the Hogan Personnel Selection Series" (Hogan and Hogan, 1986, p. 1).

Health care employees constituted a portion of the populations the Hogans researched in their reliability and validity studies. The Hogans claim that the HPSS takes about 20 to 25 minutes to complete and can be self-administered on computer-scored answer sheets. Computer-generated interpretive reports provide a nontechnical, descriptive appraisal.

Technique 3: The Expert Selection Program

The Expert Selection Program (ESP) offered by Murman (1985) is different from the HPSS in that it focuses on the interview and depends on the reliable use of validated interview questions for its results. It requires a reasonably good system of job analysis and performance documentation and skilled interviewers. Its guiding principle is that profiles of successful performers can be created on the basis of the behaviors of high-performing job incumbents. Of necessity, the distinction between high and low performers must be evidenced.

By using performance information along with job analyses, performance analyses, and managers' input, the program establishes probing questions designed to determine which applicants have behaviors similar to those found in high-performing job incumbents. The type of interview that is developed under this program requires approximately 30 to 45 minutes to conduct and can be customized to include computer-assisted scoring when interviewers are appropriately and adequately trained. Measurement Systems Corporation, the firm Murman founded, offers computer-aided scoring. You may also obtain complete interview transcription services, scoring services, and profiles of individual candidates. Alternatively, you may purchase the profiler program for personal computer application. The computer-generated profile reports are nontechnical and include graphic results in the areas of behavior identified as critical to successful performance.

Technique 4: Competency Profile

The Competency Profile technique was described by Hendrickson in 1987. Like Murman, Hendrickson believes that a "competency model can be constructed through research on high-performing job incumbents" and systematic application of the results in the assessment process (Hendrickson, 1987, p. 71). Hendrickson argues that the model is most effective when used with job categories that have the most significant impact on business objectives. As with Murman's instrument, the user must be capable of identifying high performers, collecting data describing their performance, and analyzing the data for patterns or a "blueprint of the skills, traits and motives that make a difference between outstanding and average performance in a particular job" (Hendrickson, 1987, p. 72).

Significantly, Hendrickson also points out that the sophistication of the model may vary depending on the use of external consultants and the level of statistical analysis. What is crucial in the use of a technique such as this one and like Murman's system is the *process* it suggests: a deliberate scrutiny of (1) the work to be done, (2) the environment in which it occurs, and (3) the interpersonal skills and technical competencies required for success, all of which are translated to a set of hiring objectives against which hiring and retention performance can be substantively measured.

Once the competency model has been created, an interview is constructed that is similar to the one used in Murman's system. The interview is analyzed, and the frequencies of competencies are graphed or scored in relation to the desired level of competencies. If funds are available, special computer programming support from consultants will likely permit computerized scoring and reporting.

Technique 5: Functional Assessment and Instructional Resource Program

As described by Gilbert (1978), the Functional Assessment and Instructional Resource (FAIR) program requires relatively elaborate preparation, although it is likely that most of what is required is already in place in large organizations. The necessary elements would probably be currently arranged in an organization as job descriptions, task assignments, orientation and training guides, and the like. With modifications and rearrangements, Gilbert's model might be appropriate and applicable.

Gilbert (1978, p. 325) asserts that FAIR has as its sole objective the "selection of people most likely to be exemplary performers in a specific job." According to him, "anyone can enter a FAIR program. All entrants must be given the opportunity to know the job intimately and must be given a description of what they must learn to master the job and then be given the opportunity to learn it." Further, he says that in FAIR, behavior is evaluated only when entrants have shown a mastery of the job (Gilbert, 1978, p. 326).

According to Gilbert, FAIR proceeds on the basis of a learner-guided instruction manual prepared by the hiring manager, human resources professional, or both. The manual must describe the accountabilities, requirements, performance measures, and standards for the job. Further, the manual should include a description of the theoretical basis for the work, factors distinguishing exemplary from mediocre performance, specific knowledge requirements, and a series of performance tasks designed to elicit desired performance and seal the necessary learning. Finally, the manual should specify helpful resources. A supervisor or manager must be available to oversee actual performance and to acknowledge actual accomplishments.

Final decisions about the candidates are made by a "worthy performance ratio" that gives points for job accomplishments and subtracts points for the amount of additional training an entrant required after completing the learner-guided instruction phase (Gilbert, 1978, p. 328). Unfortunately, Gilbert does not offer examples of the calculation of this ratio.

This conceptual framework may be worthy of pursuit if accelerated development for promotion or cross-training of several people becomes necessary (Manzini and Gridley, 1986). Further, this approach, or some form of it, might be exceedingly well suited to certain highly defined jobs. Theoretically, this approach might be more appropriately called a job trial. A rather elaborate series of steps seems necessary to prepare the learner-guided manual. However, the discipline such preparation might impose could result in greater effectiveness in analyzing the work to be done in a given area and therefore could result in greater effectiveness in selecting employees for the area. Perhaps the most disconcerting factor associated with this technique is the perceived amount of time required for the preparation and assessment.

Technique 6: Assessment Centers

According to Feuer and Lee (1988, p. 24), "An assessment center is not a place. Rather, it is a method for predicting on-the-job behavior." An assessment center is different from the other techniques presented in this chapter because it makes use of multiple assessment techniques, at least one of which is a job-related simulation. In an assessment center, a group of persons come together for one or more days to act as assessors who appraise several individuals at a time. The assessment center also standardizes the methods for making inferences from the techniques. It is likely to predict performance successfully because, as Cascio (1982) has suggested, it pools the judgments of multiple assessors in rating each candidate's behavior.

However, assessment centers are expensive. Feuer and Lee (1988, p. 25) have pointed out that "not only does a company have to analyze jobs and construct exercises and job simulations, it must also train employees or supervisors familiar with the job to act as assessors. That's one of the reasons it's a technique that has been largely reserved for either selecting managers or pinpointing their training and development needs."

However, a growing number of large companies are adapting assessment center methods for the assessment and selection of blue-collar workers. This is especially true in the companies with Japanese ties. In these firms, there is a concept known as *kaizen* — which Feuer and Lee (1988, p. 23) say is defined by Masaaki Imai, a Japanese author, as a "deeply ingrained Japanese value that says everything deserves to be constantly, patiently, incrementally improved." Feuer and Lee further say that people like GenCorp's Ray Casper, director of human resources, fully embrace *kaizen* as a concept by which to govern their operations. To hire the "right stuff" for such an environment of incessant, constant searches for improvement requires more than "an application, a back X ray, and a few reference calls." Thus, say Feuer and Lee (1988, p. 24), more companies are using assessment center technologies. "These firms put every applicant — from entry-level production worker through the general manager — through what most would consider an arduous selection procedure. Applicants are screened not only for technical skills and aptitudes but for attitudes that will allow them to flourish in a team environment."

Many large hospitals have instituted assessment centers, especially for the purposes of selecting or developing nurse managers. A few have widened the use of the concept to include other management positions. Some organizations inevitably will consider or implement this technique of selection and development of key positions throughout their organizations, whether or not those positions are in management.

Small hospitals may have difficulty finding the resources for such an effort. Nevertheless, some kind of consortia might be possible when certain hospitals can determine that competitive forces would not negate cooperation in such an effort. Small, independent rural hospitals that have established relationships with tertiary care centers might pursue the idea of cooperation in assessment centers.

In addition to the writers cited in this section, two others should be mentioned. George Thornton and William Byham (1982) offer important scholarly and thorough work on the subject of assessment centers. Study of their analyses should be helpful to those considering the technique.

Conclusion

At the beginning of this chapter, I presented a theoretical case study. I asked several questions about how you would run a business so clearly troubled with serious problems.

All the questions I posed could have been reduced to three simple ones: What is next? Who else besides us is worrying about the future? How can we prevent even worse things than the headaches we have today?

When Odiorne (1981, pp. 220–21) asks these questions, he answers, "Anticipatory management." He compellingly and powerfully challenges us to remember that the "joys of anticipation often exceed the pleasures of realization." "Furthermore," he says, "the realization of a planned and consciously chosen objective will exceed that of the random or surprise success. Management by anticipation substitutes planned change for joy rides."

In this context, if you are now in a situation in which you feel total satisfaction with the way your assessment and selection system is working, anticipate for a moment how far the current state of affairs will carry your organization into its future. Anticipate when the demands of your organization might necessitate a change in methods. If you are dissatisfied with this aspect of your organization, anticipate what sorts of things you would encounter daily if you achieved the state where you would be satisfied.

Over the long run, says Odiorne, this way of approaching life has numerous rewards. Among them are the following:

- Chaos is reduced.
- Personal stress from unintended consequences is minimized.
- A wide basis of participation from subordinates is provided when job-related decisions will affect them.
- The freedom to decide what should happen and the latitude to make it happen are gratifying and replace waiting for something to happen to us.
- The sense of powerlessness and meaninglessness that sometimes invades an organization and its people decreases substantially.

Odiorne speculates that this anticipatory approach actually engenders optimism, which he says has the dimension of being a self-fulfilling prophecy when it permeates an organization. In this work, Odiorne clearly reminds us that people really do want to be splendid and shining. Another writer, Robert Waterman (1987), says that renewing organizations and the renewers within them create an incessant optimism.

Maslow (1971, p. 53) talked about renewal in this way:

We are not in a position in which we have nothing to work with. We already have a start; we already have capacities, talents, direction, missions, callings. The job is, if we are willing to take it seriously, to help ourselves to be more perfectly what we already are, to be more full, more actualizing, more realizing, in fact what we are in potentiality.

What better time do we have than now to produce work that creates optimism? What better opportunity is there to enhance assessment and selection to ensure that the hope and spirit so sorely needed in the health care industry are born into its ranks? Imaginative consideration of the systems and techniques through which candidates are assessed and selected commands the attention of the human resources profession and all managers concerned with the success of our enterprises. Consummating and documenting successful improvements in this aspect of our work endows our companies with stamina, balance, and confidence.

References

Arvey, R. D. *Fairness in Selecting Employees.* Reading, MA: Addison-Wesley Publishing Co., 1979.

Arvey, R. D., and Campion, J. E. The employment interview: a summary and review of recent research. *Personnel Psychology* 35:281–322, 1982.

Bureau of National Affairs. *Recruiting and Selection Procedures.* Personnel Policies Forum Survey No. 146. Washington, DC: Bureau of National Affairs, 1988, pp. 17–19.

Cascio, W. F. *Costing Human Resources: The Financial Impact of Behavior in Organizations.* New York City: Van Nostrand Reinhold Company, 1982.

Center for Health Policy Research, Oklahoma Medical Research Foundation. *Uncompensated Care and Rural Hospitals.* Oklahoma City: Oklahoma City Chamber of Commerce, 1988, p. 18.

Feuer, D., and Lee, C. The kaizen connection: how companies pick tomorrow's workers. *Training* 25(5):23–35, May 1988.

Garfield, C. *Peak Performers: The New Heroes of American Business.* New York City: William Morrow and Co., 1986, pp. 35–38.

Gilbert, T. F. *Human Competence: Engineering Worthy Performance.* New York City: McGraw-Hill Book Co., 1978.

Hendrickson, J. Hiring the "right stuff." *Personnel Administrator* 32(11):70–74, Nov. 1987.

Hogan, J., and Hogan, R. *Hogan Personnel Selection Series™ Manual.* Tulsa: University of Tulsa, 1986.

Hogan, R. Development of an empathy scale. *Journal of Consulting and Clinical Psychology* 33:307–16, 1969.

Manzini, A. O., and Gridley, J. D. *Integrating Human Resources and Strategic Business Planning.* New York City: AMACOM (American Management Association), 1986.

Maslow, A. *The Farther Reaches of Human Nature.* New York City: Viking Press, 1971.

Murman, M. A Proposal for Creating a System of Selecting High Performing Employees. Unpublished. Lincoln, NE: Measurement Systems, 1985, pp. 5–11.

Odiorne, G. S. *The Change Resisters.* Englewood Cliffs, NJ: Prentice-Hall, 1981.

Rubin, R. J., Moran, D. W., Jones, K. S., and Hachboren, M. A. *Critical Condition— America's Healthcare in Jeopardy.* Washington, DC: Lewin/ICF (a division of Health and Sciences Research, Inc.), 1988.

Thornton, G. C., III, and Byham, W. C. *Assessment Centers and Managerial Performance.* New York City: Academic Press, 1982.

Waterman, R. H., Jr. *The Renewal Factor: How the Best Get and Keep the Competitive Edge.* New York City: Bantam Books, 1987.

Chapter 7

Performance Management Systems

James A. Landry

Introduction

Evaluating the performance of other people is not unique to the 20th century. Passing judgment has always been and conceivably always will be a phenomenon of human social behavior. For example, the emperors of the Wei dynasty in China (A.D. 221–265) had an imperial rater whose task it was to evaluate the performance of the royal family. Ignatius Loyola established a system for the formal seating of members of the Jesuit Society. And Robert Owen of Scotland devised the first-recorded appraisal system in industry by placing a colored block at each workman's place to designate how well the worker had performed the previous day (different colors indicated various levels of performance).

Formal appraisals were first used in the United States by the federal government and some city administrations in the early 1900s. Frederick Taylor laid the groundwork for the use of performance appraisals in business and industry with his work measurement program. After World War I, several performance appraisal techniques that focused on personality and behavioral traits came into use. However, it was not until the early 1950s that work-oriented qualities began to be integrated into the performance appraisal techniques of American business and government.

Since the 1950s, the types, approaches, and uses of performance appraisals have grown dramatically. Behavioral scientists, human resources professionals, executives, collective bargaining constituents, bureaucrats, legal experts, and industrial engineers — as well as employees whose sentiments and, at times, input have been considered — have contributed significantly to the development and improvement of existing methodologies.

With the proliferation of performance appraisal techniques, there is a need for a performance management system that allows managers to select techniques appropriate to the organization and to utilize these techniques correctly, systematically, flexibly, and continually. To explain what is meant by the use of the term *system,* this chapter will begin by examining the variety of outcomes that organizations expect from their approaches to performance management and the larger frame of reference (the gestalt) in which performance management activities take place. From this examination, it should become clear that no single technique can achieve the variety of outcomes that management legitimately desires.

Management Expectations of Performance Management

Organizations continue to commit resources to the improvement of the performance measurement process because they recognize that a good methodology can and will improve performance. Furthermore, organizations realize that in order to function and grow, they must implement some kind of periodic performance assessment to ensure that every part of the organization meets output objectives within quality specifications and with the optimum use of the resources available and to ensure that the maximum growth of personnel, in job knowledge and skills, is achieved.

At face value these goals might seem easily achievable, but organizations continue to be perplexed in finding the most effective performance measurement tools. Performance management systems are expected to ensure adequate performance and development while simultaneously appraising performance fairly and objectively, communicating the appraisal so that it is understood and appreciated, and turning the total process into a motivator for improved performance. Little has changed over the years as to what management expects or at least hopes for from performance appraisals. Managers still want appraisals to identify marginal behavior, aid employee development, assess an employee's potential for advancement, and act as a valid defense in discrimination suits. However, as in days gone by, the controversy continues as to which system is best.

Traditional versus Collaborative Approaches

As a result of the considerable time and effort organizations have spent in designing, implementing, monitoring, and defending the performance appraisal process, two primary approaches have emerged. The first is the traditional approach, which is quantitative and statistical in design (for example, scalar ranking, such as when a supervisor appraises an employee's performance according to a scale of one to five). The second is the collaborative approach, which emphasizes communicating, matching expectations between supervisor and subordinate, and setting goals (for example, management by objectives). When the scope of the job is limited and employees do not have a strong need for feedback and development, the traditional approach works well. In jobs in which varied and flexible decision making is necessary, however, employees with a high need for achievement will be more satisfied with a collaborative approach to performance appraisal.

What has occurred, in part, as a result of these two approaches is an organizational neurosis. That is, the organization may experience dissatisfaction with its present appraisal methodology, may realize that something needs to be changed, and may even be aware of alternatives for change; but the organization fears moving away from what is known and predictable (the current approach) to something unknown and therefore less predictable (a new approach). This dilemma may result in indecision; thus, the organization remains frustrated. The organization may want a collaborative approach that will help people grow and develop, and yet the organization may perceive it to be necessary to use a traditional approach that can withstand external challenges such as governmental scrutiny and legal action. In addition, the traditional approach may seem less cumbersome to administer and manage.

Whatever approach(es) the organization chooses to implement as a means of evaluating performance, they will significantly affect the results of the organization (that is, goals and objectives) as well as the needs and efforts of its employees. If, on the one hand, ambiguity, deception, or both are found in the performance appraisal methodology, the neurosis will be exacerbated and will invariably result in high levels of anxiety and poor results. If, on the other hand, performance assessments are meaningful, tied to job responsibilities, understood by employees, used as the basis for fair rewards, and linked to the organization's business goals and objectives, any neurotic tendencies will be kept in balance. The organization should experience positive movement if realistic organizational objectives have been established and effectively meshed with the performance management system.

Productivity and Performance

Productivity should not be confused with or misconstrued as performance. Although often used interchangeably, the two terms are defined differently. *Productivity* is a measure of the efficiency and effectiveness with which an organization turns out goods and services. *Effectiveness* is doing the right things at the right times, and *efficiency* is the ratio of output per unit of input. For example, the productivity of the nursing department could be defined in terms of quality of care (effectiveness) and how cost-efficiently the care was delivered (efficiency). Productivity does not mean working harder and faster. It does mean working smarter.

Performance means the actual accomplishment or completion of one's goals, objectives, duties, or responsibilities, as distinguished from potential ability, capacity, knowledge, skills, or aptitude to do so. Performance appraisal methodologies are techniques or tools to enhance or improve productivity. They are vehicles to assist employees to work smarter because performance appraisal takes into account those factors that influence productivity.

In health care, a productivity (output) measurement represents quality of care expressed, for example, by rates of morbidity, rates of mortality, or levels of wellness at discharge at a reasonable cost. Declines in manpower (for example, nursing shortages) and increases in the costs associated with materials, salaries, and operating expenditures are factors, or inputs, that affect productivity. Performance criteria based on these inputs, preferably objective and measurable criteria, are established to enhance the efficiency and effectiveness of the predicted or expected outputs.

Pay for Performance

In mid-1987, the Wyatt Company conducted a special survey of more than 800 U.S. companies, including more than 100 health care institutions, in which company representatives were asked various questions concerning pay for performance—how well it is supported by management, how well the performance management system rewards performance, how performance is measured, and what the major problems are with regard to implementing pay for performance. The results of the survey suggested five major points.

First, companies were generally dissatisfied with their performance management systems. Only 31 percent of the responding companies rated their present salary administration programs as successful in relating pay to performance (figure 7-1).

Second, the pay for performance concept was a high priority in most companies. All management/supervisory groups showed strong interest in the concept. Fifty-six percent of top-level managers and 66 percent of human resources managers rated it a very high priority (table 7-1).

Third, the major impediments to the overall success of pay for performance systems were:

1. Inadequate training of managers (mentioned by 55 percent of the respondents)
2. Lack of objective measurement (40 percent)
3. Not enough money (39 percent)
4. Poor system administration and design (27 percent)

Fourth, the major impediments to successful ratings were:

1. Inconsistent ratings (59 percent)
2. Too much subjectivity in the rating procedure (54 percent)

Figure 7-1. Success of Present Salary Administration Program in Recognizing Pay for Performance

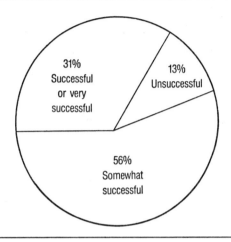

31%
Successful
or very
successful

13%
Unsuccessful

56%
Somewhat
successful

Source: The Wyatt Company (1987).

Table 7-1. Perceptions of Commitment to Pay for Performance (Rated as a Very High Priority by Respondents)

Respondents	Percentage
Human resources staff	66
Top-level management	56
Middle-level management	35
Immediate supervisors	25
Exempt employees	21

Source: The Wyatt Company (1987).

3. Inadequately trained supervisors (52 percent)
4. Too many high ratings (48 percent)

(Table 7-2 lists these and other impediments.)

Fifth, nearly two thirds of the responding companies were considering changes in their programs to improve pay for performance (table 7-3).

The findings of the survey, in general, showed a combination of dissatisfaction and hope: Few were satisfied with their current program, but most planned to make improvements. The plans focused on training and communication but may result in continuing frustration if not designed and implemented by the interdisciplinary efforts of those representing the necessary spectrum of functional areas.

Table 7-2. Major Problems with Current Performance Appraisal Systems

Problems	Percentage
Inconsistencies in ratings	59
Too much subjectivity	54
Poorly trained supervisors	52
Rating inflation	48
Supervisors manipulate ratings	35
Too many employees rated in the middle	25
Obsolete rating procedures	14
System too complicated/not accepted	12
Forced curve	8
Other	8

Source: The Wyatt Company (1987).

Table 7-3. Improvements Considered for or Made in Pay for Performance Programs

Improvement	Percentage
Redesign of appraisal system	43
Increased management training	39
Redesign of policies/procedures	30
Improved communication	28
Tighter controls	23
Individual/group incentives	19
Top-level management support	16
One-time special awards	16
Other	10

Source: The Wyatt Company (1987).

Performance Management: The Gestalt

Whatever method management uses to guide performance and increase productivity, there will be a requirement inherent in the organization's culture for a systematic way to direct the organization's activities. Therefore, the organization must be appreciated and respected as a complex whole composed of interactive and dynamic parts (that is, the gestalt). An organization has a mission that is directly related to the product it produces or the service it delivers. To carry out its mission effectively and efficiently, it must consider its structure, people, resources, policies, and technology.

In addition, every organization experiences ongoing change as a result of the dynamic fluctuations or adjustments within or between one or more of its parts. Mergers and acquisitions probably are the most dramatic kind of change an organization can experience; a change of chief executive officer, the organization's steward, may be a close second. Changes in federal policy that could affect organizational policy, advances in technology that could eliminate existing jobs or create new ones, and appearances of collective bargaining units that could reorganize segments of the work force are among other potential changes with far-reaching consequences.

The performance management system (PMS) is one part of the organization's gestalt, but the PMS part has a gestalt of its own because it, too, is composed of parts (for example, philosophy, nonfinancial rewards, and incentives). (See figure 7-2.) The meaning, intent, and effectiveness of the PMS is derived from the interactiveness within the PMS's whole and the dynamic interplay between the PMS's whole and the organization's whole (gestalt).

Figure 7-2. PMS and the Organization's Gestalt

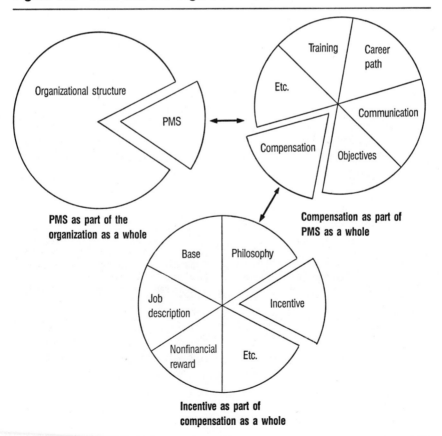

Like the organization, the PMS experiences change as a result either of alterations within its own subparts (for example, the introduction of a new compensation strategy—gainsharing) or of organizational changes (for example, the hiring of a new director of human resources who has different ideas about performance measurement).

Change can cause many things to happen. It can create opportunity and positive direction or stifle and inhibit growth; it can offer new or additional choices or create further dependency; it can fulfill dreams or curb ambitions. Whatever change brings, it is always accompanied by tension and anxiety, because it represents movement into less experienced, less known, and less predictable areas. Anxiety is the gap between now and later. The less employees know, understand, and accept changes in the PMS, the higher is the level of anxiety.

In any organizational gestalt, the organization is looking for closure, that is, closing the gap between now and later and thereby reducing feelings of tension and anxiety. Thus, to be successful the PMS (or any part of the organization, for that matter) must be understood and, to the extent possible, appreciated by the employees. The closer an organization can get to reaching closure and thus becoming complete and whole, the more productive and efficient it will become and remain.

Performance Management: System versus Technique

The system of performance management often is confused with the techniques of performance appraisal. The focus in this discussion is on the effectiveness of the performance management system rather than on the strengths and weaknesses of various appraisal techniques. Many good appraisal forms and techniques have been developed (tables 7-4 and 7-5), but they must be

Table 7-4. Methods of Performance Appraisal

Rating Method	Lead to Valid Pay Decisions	Develop Employee	Improve Employee/ Supervisor Communication	Link with Organizational Planning	Involve Employee in Own Work Planning
Trait-rating scales	Low/medium	Low	Low	Low	Low
BARS	High	Medium	Medium	Low	Low
Work standards/ responsibilities	Medium	Medium	Medium	Low	Low
Management by objectives	Medium	Medium/high	High	High	High
Hybrid	Medium/high	High	High	High	High

Table 7-5. Cost of Measurement Methods

Rating Method	Development (creating the method, forms, and so forth)	Introduction (training managers and employees)	Maintenance (management time and revision costs)
Trait-rating scales	Low	Low	Low
BARS	High	Low	Medium/low
Work standards/ responsibilities	Medium	Medium	Medium
Management by objectives	Low	High	High
Hybrid	Medium	High	High

properly developed and correctly used if accurate performance assessments are to be made. The effectiveness of a generally useful technique, such as behaviorally anchored rating scales (BARS), can be compromised by a poorly designed performance management system.

For example, a good performance management system does not combine an employee's performance evaluation meeting with a salary review meeting. If they are done at the same time, the employee will undoubtedly be preoccupied with whether he or she is going to get a raise. The employee will have virtually no interest in the appraisal methodology, in this case BARS, and any opportunity for effective performance counseling and coaching will be lost. (See the next section of this chapter for a discussion of these principles.)

The performance management system parallels what has been described as performance planning. It is a dynamic, results-oriented process that enables employees and managers to continually evaluate progress against predetermined targets. It provides enough flexibility for adjustments or other changes. It ensures ongoing communication and improves morale and productivity by encouraging employees. It focuses attention more on the future than on the past. An effective PMS should transcend the static atmosphere created by using techniques alone. For instance, a technique would be using an annual box-checking exercise that appraises abstract personality traits, followed by a frustrating and uncomfortable diagnostic consultation.

Techniques, however, are easier to manage because they are separate by nature and lack the complexities and intricacies of a system. As such, techniques can be and often are stand-alone products designed to assist with management efficiencies; but they fall short, at times, in assisting with management effectiveness. A system, on the other hand, can be more effective, and efficiencies will be gained through the appropriate selection of the techniques employed in building the system.

Performance Management System Structure

The success or failure of any system, including that of a performance management system (table 7-6), depends on the balance between process and technique.

Balancing Process with Technique

The *process* of performance management involves three major activities: planning and developing, implementing and monitoring, and evaluating and realigning.

- *Planning and developing:* Employees ask themselves where they are and where they want to go.
- *Implementing and monitoring:* Once employees are where they want to go, they ask themselves how it feels and whether it really is where they want to be.
- *Evaluating and realigning:* Employees ask themselves what they can change to make their present stage of attainment even better.

Table 7-6. Key Reasons for Success and Failure of PMS

Success	Failure
• PMS is an integral part of organization's management strategy and business plan.	• PMS lacks support from top-level management. Appraisal techniques are weighted toward subjective rather than objective quantifiable factors.
• PMS is supported by top-level management.	
• The philosophy, purpose, and objectives of organization are clearly stated so that PMS can be designed to reflect these.	• PMS fails to recognize individual differences in job duties and responsibilities.
• The purposes, policies, and procedures of PMS are identified, communicated, and understood by all employees.	• PMS emphasizes past performances.
	• PMS lacks clarity and understanding as to how PMS outcomes are to be used, for example, pay raises and career development.
• A clear relationship exists between job responsibilities and performance measures.	• Evaluators/appraisers are poorly trained in areas such as coaching and counseling subordinates, giving and receiving feedback, and interviewing techniques.
• PMS is results oriented with focus on observable behavior and quantifiable objectives.	
• PMS tools are compatible with purpose for which they will be used.	• PMS is perceived as cumbersome, complex, too time-consuming, not productive, and so forth.
• Evaluators receive sufficient training on design, implementation, and evaluation of PMS.	• System is seldom reviewed.
	• System lacks overall rating consistency by evaluators.
• PMS is considered fair, equitable, and productive by participants.	• Factors have no valid correlation with good performance.
• The system is audited on a regular basis.	

This process is cyclical and constant. Employees are continually assessing their current position, which results in anticipating and calculating movement to the next and, it is hoped, better position.

Appropriate *techniques* of performance management emanate from the process and include specific tools for evaluating the process. The techniques are associated with five key factors:

- *Quantifiable:* This factor is determined by retrospective assessment as compared with data about past occurrences, prospective expectations, and how fulfillment of expectations will be measured. If an organization has acceptable data about what has happened in the past, the data should be used as a basis for what should be done in the future.
- *Operational:* This factor ensures that the responsibilities of the job are compatible with expected performance results and the organization's mission.
- *Verifiable:* This factor involves the validation and substantiation that what should occur and is expected to occur is realistic and actually does occur.
- *Acceptable:* This factor is determined by the concept that communication provides efficiency and effectiveness through understanding and appreciation.
- *Constructive:* This factor involves the identification of specific opportunities for growth, development, and enrichment.

Process implies ambiguity, activity, movement, and involvement; technique conveys specificity, measurement, and assurance. Assuming that there is good balance between the two, a meaningful organizational process focused on measurable objectives will generate appropriate techniques to measure required outcomes. Quick-fix solutions usually bypass the process and go straight to the technique. The end result, typically, is bewilderment as to why the system is not working, followed by a speedy change to a different system.

As important as process is, organizations can and often do spend too much time on it. The results of excessive focusing on process can be confounding, frustrating, and unproductive. The organization may find itself unable to act because of its indecisiveness and may thus be unable to gain the necessary impetus to take a proper course of action. Similarly, an organization can create a sense of tremendous motion by focusing on process, but the motion will be virtually out of control. An example is a hospital that is continually assessing its position in the marketplace but never takes action unless that action is a reaction.

If the organization is convinced that people want to participate in the events that affect them and will improve themselves and those around them as a result of their participation, a balance between process and technique

Figure 7-3. Development of PMS Objectives and Linkage with Organization

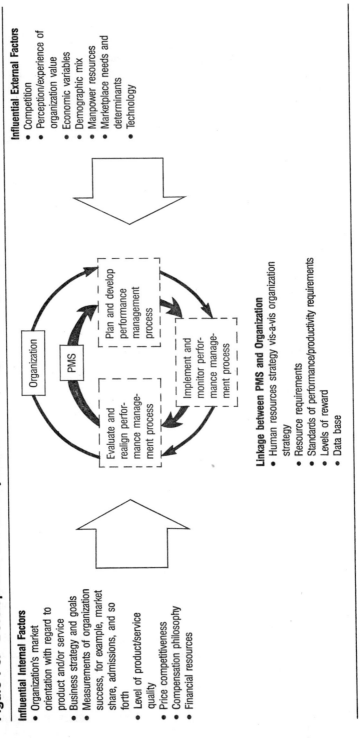

Influential External Factors
- Competition
- Perception/experience of organization value
- Economic variables
- Demographic mix
- Manpower resources
- Marketplace needs and determinants
- Technology

Organization

PMS

Plan and develop performance management process

Implement and monitor performance management process

Evaluate and realign performance management process

Linkage between PMS and Organization
- Human resources strategy vis-a-vis organization strategy
- Resource requirements
- Standards of performance/productivity requirements
- Levels of reward
- Data base

Influential Internal Factors
- Organization's market orientation with regard to product and/or service
- Business strategy and goals
- Measurements of organization success, for example, market share, admissions, and so forth
- Level of product/service quality
- Price competitiveness
- Compensation philosophy
- Financial resources

can be achieved and an appropriate performance management system for the organization can emerge. Unless the opportunity for actual involvement and input by employees is built into the system, however, too much process or too much technique will prevail.

In addition to the balancing of process with technique both within the PMS and between the organization and the PMS, the development and success of the PMS is highly dependent on the organization's ability to perceive, understand, and react well to the internal and external factors influencing the organization (figure 7-3). Although the organizational shell shields the PMS to a large degree, the shell can be permeated and, therefore, put in a position of reaction to change caused by the infringement of one or more factors. The organization must be able to employ the PMS to deal with internal and external factors by deflecting injurious, hostile, or negative forces and by taking advantage of opportunities and profiting by them.

Key Objectives, Considerations, and Questions

In developing, implementing, and evaluating any performance management system, certain key objectives, considerations, and questions should be considered (figures 7-4 and 7-5 and table 7-7). Among them are the following:

- Translating organizational goals into specific objectives for individuals
- Identifying performance requirements necessary to accomplish overall objectives of the position

Figure 7-4. Key Objectives for the Performance Management System

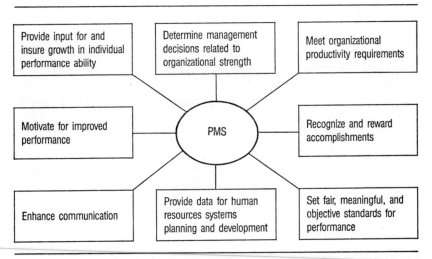

Figure 7-5. Key Considerations for a Performance Management System

Planning and Development

Quantifiable

- Decide on work expectations—what should be carried out.
- Determine measurement requirements—develop meaningful and realistic objectives and measures for performance.
- Emphasize past experience, future performance, or both.
- Analyze organization's commitment to and desire for a pay for performance system or merit system and identify organizational, unit (department), and individual measures that depend on varying conditions and environments.
- Evaluate overall competitiveness.

Operational

- Review compensation philosophy and determine compensation objectives—decision to lead or lag the market (that is, offer more money to new employees than others are offering, or offer less while depending on benefits to attract new employees), method of appraisal, affordability of plan, and so forth.
- Ensure sufficient flexibility for management discretion to accommodate changes in strategy, structure, and people.
- Ensure that performance targets are related to the requirements of the job.
- Ensure that individual objectives and goals are applicable and tied to business plan.
- Ensure that the performance assessments are linked to salary administration program.
- Ensure that the employee has a clear, consistent understanding of job function.
- Ensure that the system meets legal requirements, including legislation covering civil rights, affirmative action, and discrimination.
- Consider ease of administration while allowing for flexibility to adjust program's specifics on the basis of changes in business objectives, external factors, or both.

Verifiable

- Plan performance improvement and personal growth goals.
- Determine measurement frequency.
- Stage action plans for key results.
- Review performance requirements with incumbents to clarify task as well as quantity or quality performance criteria.

Acceptable

- Devise communication strategies—employees must know how system works.
- Explain job functions and performance requirements to managers, supervisors, and employees.
- Gain commitment from employees by involving employees in planning.

Constructive

- Make sure that the PMS is integrated with other organizational processes and is not treated as a stand-alone activity.
- Consider the organization's demands versus the employees' needs—address what is expected, how employees are doing, where they are going, how they can improve, what the reward is for doing a good job or an excellent job.
- Prepare clear, measurable standards resulting in measurement of productivity rather than activity.
- Discern differences between performance and development needs.
- Ensure commitment by management.
- Identify time horizons in meeting objectives, that is, 6 months, quarterly, annually.
- Make PMS a tool rather than a management task.
- Provide competitive rewards.

Figure 7-5. Continued

Implementation and Monitoring

Quantifiable

- Prepare written, formal policies and procedures and fully documented forms.
- Ensure that evaluations conducted are consistent with established organizational standards.
- Use PMS to systematize the management of work.

Operational

- Train employees in human relations (people) skills (communication, planning, coaching, giving and receiving feedback) as well as in the rationale and mechanics of the PMS.
- Prepare a training manual, including topics such as observing performance, documenting performance, giving feedback, completing forms, and preparing for appraisal discussion.

Verifiable

- Conduct regular performance reviews.
- Make ongoing revisions as necessary and in accordance with the PMS design.

Acceptable

- Train employees in fundamental concepts that must be understood in order to make the PMS an effective management tool.
- Provide feedback through interim reports.
- Reinforce positive performance; modify negative performance.
- Involve employees in the system to obtain greater confidence in the system, have it viewed as fair, and provide greater opportunity to strengthen genuine commitment to the success of the PMS.

Constructive

- Answer questions about how employees are doing and where they are going.
- Help supervisors observe employees more closely and do a better job of evaluating.
- Spot new training needs.
- Correct planning mistakes before it is too late.
- Be ready with suggested action steps for solving problems.

Evaluation and Realignment

Quantifiable

- Analyze reasons for success or failure.
- Conduct an annual systems audit.
- Provide backup data for management decisions that answer questions about merit increases, promotion, demotion, and termination.

Operational

- Modify job description(s) and corresponding performance measures as necessary.

Verifiable

- Analyze the organization's goals and objectives measured against performance results and determine appropriateness of the PMS to the organization's mission.

Acceptable

- Solicit input/feedback (focus group, questionnaire, and so forth) from employees to determine effectiveness and level of satisfaction with the PMS.

Constructive

- Adjust program specifics on the basis of changes in business objectives, external factors, or both.
- Recognize individual performance contributions by rewarding individual results.

- Ask whether the assessment of performance contributes to the organization's mission.
- Identify the organization's strengths and weaknesses.
- Recognize employees for their accomplishments.

Table 7-7. Key Questions for PMS Planning and Development

Quantifiable	Operational	Verifiable	Acceptable	Constructive
		Planning and Development		
Organizational: What are meaningful and realistic objectives and measures of performance for the organization?	*Organizational:* What are the compensation philosophy and, likewise, compensation objectives, as depicted in organization's salary administration program?	*Organizational:* How will we verify what is expected is appropriate, accurate, and effectively and efficiently measured?	*Organizational:* What communication strategies will be employed to ensure that the system works?	*Organizational:* Is there a commitment by management to totally integrate PMS into the organizational process and mission?
Employee: What level of performance is expected of me?	*Employee:* Are the performance measurements related to my job description and integrated with its primary functions?	*Employee:* What type of performance appraisal will be used?	*Employee:* What say do I have in determining whether the performance management system realistically measures effectiveness in doing my job and, in turn, provides meaningful incentives to do better?	*Employee:* What's in this for me?
		Implementation and Monitoring		
Organizational: What policies, procedures, and forms will we use to systematize the management of work?	*Organizational:* What training methodology will we use to ensure acceptance and understanding as well as commitment to PMS?	*Organizational:* Do managers relinquish any authority by involving subordinates in the PMS process?	*Organizational:* How do we best reinforce positive performance and modify negative performance in an ongoing way?	*Organizational:* How do we correct any planning mistakes before it's too late?

		Evaluation and Realignment		
Employee: When, where, and how often will my performance be reviewed?	*Employee:* Is there anything I should do in preparing for my review?	*Employee:* What happens if I'm in complete disagreement with the appraisal?	*Employee:* How will I receive feedback on how I'm doing?	*Employee:* How can I improve for the future?
Organizational: What is the impact of the PMS on the quality, quantity, cost, and output of our product?	*Organizational:* How do we effectively analyze the reasons for success or failure of the PMS?	*Organizational:* What is the relationship between management, supervisory, and employee involvement in the PMS d3sign?	*Organizational:* How do we best maximize outcomes of the PMS to overcome organizational weaknesses, capitalize on strengths, and maximize opportunities?	*Organizational:* How do we best adjust the PMS on the basis of changes in the organization's business objectives, external factors, or both?
Employee: How did I do?	*Employee:* Will there be any changes in my job responsibilities?	*Employee:* Is my potential taken into account, or only what I've done to date?	*Employee:* Do you value my input on perforrnance requirements for this job?	*Employee:* How can I do better?

- Providing a fair, equitable, and timely evaluation of employee performance as it pertains to established measurement criteria
- Fostering communication between the supervisor and the subordinate on how the employee is progressing in comparison with expected performance results
- Improving work performance and productivity through the collaboration of the organization, managers, supervisors, and employees
- Rewarding and recognizing accomplishments in a timely and equitable manner
- Identifying the organization's strengths and weaknesses
- Motivating employees through feedback
- Providing a sound basis for salary administration actions
- Providing information to management for career planning and training
- Building mutual understanding that will encourage managers, supervisors, and employees to work together in meeting the organization's and individual's goals

Conclusion

Rating performance continues to be a necessary evil for organizations, managers, and individual employees alike. There is agreement that individual differences do exist in performance and that those differences should be acknowledged and rewarded accordingly. It makes absolute sense in theory. However, in design, implementation, and practice, it can be the most difficult and problematic issue that management faces. Issues such as identifying performance factors, criteria for measurement, the relationship and linkage of individual measures to departmental goals or the organization's vision or both, equitable and differential rewards, modes of communication and motivation, and the relationship of productivity inputs and performance outputs all require examination and reconciliation. To do so effectively requires a regard for and a sensitivity to the interplay of the organization's dynamic parts.

References

Bureau of National Affairs. *Pay for Performance in the Health Care Industry.* Washington, DC: Bureau of National Affairs, 1987, pp. 1–20.

Caruth, D., Middlebrook, B., and Rachel, F. Performance appraisals: much more than a once-a-year task. *Supervisory Management* 27(9):28–36, Sept. 1982.

Cole, E. Performance appraisal or performance measurement: which is more effective? Internal human resources publication, Marsh & McLennan Companies, New York City, pp. 1–6.

DeVries, D. L. Viewing performance appraisal with a wide angle lens. Proceedings of a symposium at American Psychological Association Convention, Aug. 1983, pp. 40–42.

Friedman, M. G. 10 steps to objective appraisals. *Personnel Journal* 65(6):66–71, June 1986.

Gutteridge, T. G., and Otte, F. L. Organizational career development: what's going on out there? *Training and Development Journal* 37(2):22–26, Feb. 1983.

Halley, W., and Field, H. Will your performance appraisal system hold up in court? *Personnel* 59(1):59–64, Jan.–Feb. 1982.

Harper, S. C. Adding purpose to performance reviews. *Training and Development Journal* 40(9):53–55, Sept. 1986.

Kury, P. *Performance Planning and Appraisal.* New York City: McGraw-Hill, 1984, p. 160.

Lawler, E. E., Mohrman, A. M., and Resnick, S. M. Performance appraisal revisited. *Organizational Dynamics* 13(1):39–54, Summer 1984.

Louergran, W. G. Coaching the coaches to coach. *The Executive,* Winter 1986, pp. 1–7.

Mannisto, M. An assessment of productivity in healthcare. *Hospitals* 54(18):71–76, Sept. 16, 1980.

Martin, D. C. Performance appraisal, 2: improving the raters' effectiveness. *Personnel* 63(8):28–33, Aug. 1986.

Olson, R. F. *Performance Appraisal: A Guide to Greater Productivity.* New York City: John Wiley & Sons, 1981, p. 191.

Richards, G. Working smarter. *Hospitals* 57(19):92–100, Oct. 1, 1983.

Romburg, R. V. Performance appraisal, 1: risks and rewards. *Personnel* 63(8):20–26, Aug. 1986.

Sashkin, M. Appraising appraisals: ten lessons from research for practice. *Organizational Dynamics* 9(3):37–50, Winter 1981.

Schneier, C. E., Beatty, R. W., and Baird, L. S. Creating a performance management system. *Training and Development Journal* 40(5):74–79, May 1986.

Schneier, C. E., Beatty, R. W., and Baird, L. S. How to construct a successful performance appraisal system. *Training and Development Journal* 40(4):38–42, Apr. 1986.

Sears, D. L. Situational performance appraisals. *Supervisory Management* 29(5):6–10, May 1984.

Taylor, R. L., and Zawacki, R. A. Trends in performance appraisal: guidelines for managers. *Personnel Administrator* 29(3):71–80, Mar. 1984.

U.S. Department of Health and Human Services. *Productivity and Health: Papers on Incentives for Improving Health Productivity.* Publication HRA 80-14025. Washington, DC: U.S. Department of Health and Human Services, pp. 1–71 [no date available].

Wells, R. G. Guidelines for effective and defensible performance appraisal systems. *Personnel Journal* 61(10):776–82, Oct. 1982.

The Wyatt Company. *The 1987 Wyatt Performance Management Survey.* Boston: The Wyatt Company, 1987.

Chapter 8

Recognition and Reward

James A. Landry

Introduction

Most people have taken an introductory psychology course that introduced them to such names as Freud, Jung, Sullivan, Maslow, Skinner, and Piaget and have come to accept or reject in total or in part psychological theories on personality development. Whether individuals agree with any one theory really does not matter. However, almost all trained theorists and amateur analysts alike seem to be in strong agreement when it comes to understanding the importance and significance of recognition and reward to personality development.

There is general agreement that humans go through stages of development. Movement through these stages solidifies the foundation of personality. A shaping of the sense of self occurs, and personal identity is crystallized. Reward and recognition are introduced from birth onward as interventions to encourage and manipulate successful achievements through continual reinforcement. People learn what is acceptable and what is not; if they meet or exceed expectations, they usually are rewarded.

Another key factor in reward and recognition is the need to satisfy or please others. Some self-contained individuals claim that they are content to let others take all the glory. Such people are few and far between; no one is completely altruistic. If people lived in a vacuum, they would be void of self-concept. People need and rely on others to give them feedback and thereby support the development of self-esteem and self-worth. People not only give others feedback through their actions and deeds, they also provide insight into possible self-improvements as well as encouragement to move forward.

Reward and recognition appear in many forms. They may be attained or obtained; that is, a person can be given something by someone else, or a person can give himself or herself something. In either case, the sentiment is that the person earned the reward and deserved it. Individual priorities and value systems determine the level of importance and the total worth of the reward or recognition received. This chapter will examine the reward and recognition mechanisms health care institutions use to address the factors just described: reinforcement of expected behavior and performance, incentives for exceeding expectations, feedback on what performance the management values, and rewards matched to employee value systems.

Reward and Recognition: A Health Care Industry Perspective

It would be an understatement to say that the health care industry has experienced many dramatic changes over the past several years. Change has been most pronounced in the fiscal area, with more interest and attention paid to the costs of services delivered and net income received—simply, the bottom line. There is a much more aggressive approach to health care cost management today than in the past, when health care was truly viewed as an entitlement, when costs did not matter because there was 100 percent company-paid coverage.

The change in management perspective toward running health care like a business has, of course, caused a tightening of the belts. New methods (new to health care, anyway) and techniques to streamline operations and gain efficiencies have been implemented. With limited budgets, many health care organizations have been forced to consider how to provide high-quality care in a cost-effective way. Pay-for-performance systems, particularly incentive and productivity models, have been designed to produce the fiscal efficiencies needed by the health care provider and to allow the secondary asset of producing employee satisfaction related to reward for effort.

As the health care industry becomes more complex to manage, with increased competition and scrutiny of costs by the public, the prevalence of incentive compensation arrangements in the future will dramatically increase. Incentive plans provide motivation for creativity, innovation, teamwork, dedication, and, most important, results. These factors seem to be important, if not absolute, requirements for success. Incentive plans today and in the future will reflect a dramatic change in the compensation philosophy of health care organizations. As illustrated by figure 8-1, we will see more emphasis on justification for pay (the *for what*) as opposed to automatic adjustments (the *how much*) or adjustments made on the basis of ill-defined, subjective appraisal criteria (the *measured how*).

Figure 8-1.   Compensation Philosophy

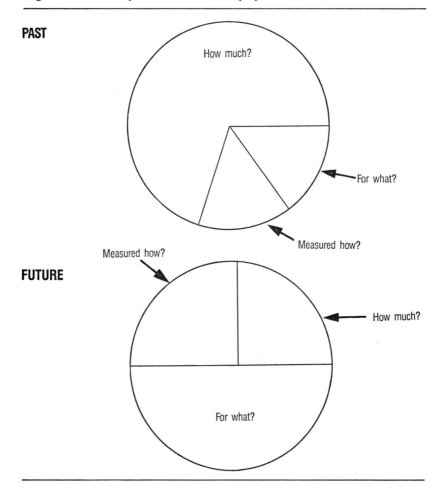

Well-thought-out objectives for a meaningful reward and recognition plan should clarify organizational goals, sharpen the focus for management and work force efforts, add significant value to the achievement of defined levels of performance, and provide a competitive spread between compensation levels within and outside the organization. With a focus on the highest-priority needs of the organization (an outcome of setting objectives for short- and long-term goals), the incentive plan should provide greater opportunity to leverage the relationship between pay and performance. The incentive plan demystifies this relationship by making very clear via measurable objectives the linkage of pay to performance. People know up front what is expected and how they will be rewarded — a classic stimulus–response paradigm. And if the rewards are viewed as significant and not merely given for ordinary achievement or entitlement, the system will work effectively, as demonstrated by improved financial strength, expanded capabilities, and increased productivity.

Motivation and Goals

Success in attaining recognition and reward is tied directly to the level of motivation and the pursuit of realistic goals. Are people motivated by goals, or do goals motivate people? The answer is that it can go either way. Some people are highly energized, and with proper channeling they can harness that energy on focused goal setting; motivation is high and the establishment of goals naturally follows. Other people carefully evaluate alternatives, set realistic goals, and then motivate themselves for the activity.

Motivation is self-energy. Although it may be influenced from the outside (for example, the coach's pep talk at halftime), it must ultimately come from within. A person must sincerely care and want something deeply to stand any chance of making it happen.

Motivation has three important aspects: amplitude, duration, and velocity. *Amplitude* measures how much someone really wants to do something. It is the power source. If someone is not doing what he or she really wants to do, the person will ultimately fail because of a low power source. *Duration* is the sustained desire to achieve a goal. Motivation requires constant energy and enough of it to go from one point to the next. *Velocity* is speed. The value of the reward compounded by individual personality style (for example, a laid-back style versus bull-in-the-china-shop style) determines the rate at which available energy is utilized in pursuit of rewards.

Goals legitimize motivation by providing logical meaning and support to activity. A goal is a straightforward statement, written or unwritten, of what the desired outcome of a specific activity will be. Diagnosis-related groups (DRGs), prospective pricing, and the continued requirements for criteria-based performance measures from the Joint Commission on Accreditation of Healthcare Organizations are prime examples of the health care industry's movement toward specified, goal-directed activity.

Many people will never reap the reward and recognition that they feel they deserve because there is an improper balance or linkage between motivation and goals. A person with low motivation and high goals may well be all talk and no action (it is not the whistle that pulls the train). Another person may be highly motivated but have too many goals. That is goal diffusion. Although this person has high energy levels, his or her energy is not usable because it is not focused on anything specific; that is, there is no systematic pursuit. A third example is the person who is all dressed up with no place to go. This person is highly motivated and has high goals, but lacks the training, skills, or information necessary to carry out an activity and thus achieve a goal.

Organizational Demands versus Individual Needs

The rewards and recognition offered by an organization to its employees must be appropriate and meaningful. Although Shakespeare wrote that "words are but empty thanks," for many people, a sincere thank you after a job well done may be all the recognition that is necessary. However, verbal expressions of thanks are usually unacceptable as the only form of reward in daily work lives. Granted, everyone likes a pat on the back and verbal recognition, but in the real work world, the stakes are higher. If the reward and recognition offered are not perceived as meaningful, they will be construed as "but empty thanks."

In the work setting, constant interplay occurs between organizational demands and individual needs. If an organization has set realistic goals compatible with its mission, if its goals are understood and appreciated by a trained and qualified work force, and if the work force is motivated by intrinsic job satisfaction and appropriate reward incentives, then success will abound. That is the best-case scenario. Too often, however, weak links between organizational goals and individual needs can lead to an organizational breakdown. When the organization is unrealistic in setting its objectives, unrealistic expectations for employees will surely follow. No matter what the reward system, results will be unsatisfactory both to the organization and to the employee. The organization will suffer on productivity measures, turnover, accidents, and the like, and individuals will experience anger, frustration, confusion, and vulnerability (expressed overtly or covertly).

When the organization sets realistic strategic objectives, it can demand specific outcomes from its work force. That is good business. When the organization takes into account employees' needs, the outcomes will be achieved more effectively and efficiently. That is better business. The interaction of both sides will generate natural and acceptable methods for encouraging results, that is, the rewards and recognition required to generate expected results.

To create the organizational momentum required to meet impending demands, the organization creates a compensation package (figure 8-2) designed to satisfy employees' needs. Like Maslow's needs hierarchy, basic needs must be satisfied first (that is, subsistence as represented by base compensation) before one can move up to another level of satisfaction, for example, noncash rewards.

Current Trends in Merit Pay

During the 1960s, cost-of-living adjustment programs gave rise to compensation systems that used step plans. The merit system of pay evolved, in part, as a reaction to the step plans (in which pay increases were automatic and not based on criteria). These step-in-grade systems were heavily tenured

Figure 8-2.   Total Compensation Package

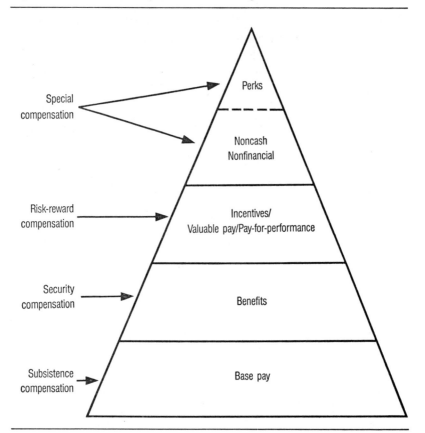

and rewards (that is, raises) were given for longevity and usually across the board (no matter what!). Step plans lack sufficient justification for pay increases other than length of service. The merit system, however, recognizes individual differences; for example, how duties are performed, how requirements are met, how people discharge their responsibilities and adjust to working conditions. A true merit system offers an opportunity to distinguish between mediocre performance and excellent performance and then pays accordingly.

Unlike true incentive pay-for-performance programs, however, merit increases usually result in increases in base pay (once an employee gets it, the employer cannot take it away). In addition, the merit system tends to relate primarily to routine organizational responsibilities. True incentive plans, on the other hand, provide variable pay in addition to the base but not added to the base. Pay varies owing to environmental factors or to the criteria that the organization values as important to meeting its mission (extrinsic) rather than to particular variances in job responsibility (intrinsic). The real incentives are also more apparent for excellent or superior performance, emphasizing stretch accomplishments. With merit systems, some employees become complacent and satisfied with pay increases associated with acceptable levels of performance — one serious drawback for such systems.

Current trends in health care (table 8-1 and figures 8-3 and 8-4) indicate a significant movement away from merit pay and toward incentive (for example, variable pay) programs for all employees. Again, this movement, in part, is somewhat reactive; organizations have realized that under the merit system, inflated performance ratings mean inflated pay increases. More significant, however, are the proactive reasons for the philosophical shift toward incentive programs:

- Incentive programs provide for meaningful differences in rewards.
- Incentive programs provide tangible, quantifiable results commensurate with organizational, departmental, and individual objectives and responsibilities.
- Incentive programs link performance, pay, and the business plan.
- Incentive programs allow greater recognition of how pay can be used to reinforce teamwork, service, and productivity improvement efforts.
- Incentive programs recognize which persons and behaviors financial rewards motivate.

Perhaps the most important reason for this shift toward incentive programs is that incentive pay is a good way to provide additional pay without increasing the base. The base is the point from which future raises and increases in benefits are derived. Given that the cost of benefits continues

Table 8-1. Incentive Plans in Health Care

Plan	Prevalence	Positions Included	Performance Period	Technique	Payment
Annual (management incentive)	Most common	Management	1 year	Target[a]	Cash
Long term (management incentive)	Less common	Top-level management	2–5 years	Performance unit[b]	Cash/stock
Productivity (organizationwide)	High interest, few nationally	All employees	Month, quarter, 6 months, year	Gainsharing[c]	Cash

[a] Each person has specific goals and has control over meeting them.
[b] Each person is awarded performance units according to his or her accomplishments, but meeting a goal depends on the efforts of several other people as well.
[c] Rewards are given to an entire department, section, or some other part of the organization on the basis of its collective performance. The rewards are divided among the employees in that department.

Figure 8-3. Movement toward Incentive Programs in Health Care

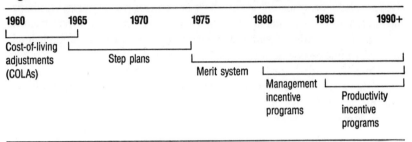

1960	1965	1970	1975	1980	1985	1990+

Cost-of-living
adjustments   Step plans
(COLAs)
                                Merit system

                                        Management
                                        incentive   Productivity
                                        programs   incentive
                                                           programs

Figure 8-4. Evolution toward Incentives

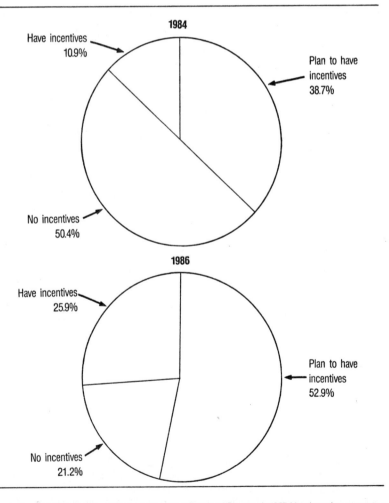

1984

Have incentives
10.9%

Plan to have
incentives
38.7%

No incentives
50.4%

1986

Have incentives
25.9%

Plan to have
incentives
52.9%

No incentives
21.2%

Source: Executive Compensation Surveys (a division of The Wyatt Company), 1987 (data based on responses from 423 health care organizations).

to escalate at an alarming rate, incentive arrangements have the advantage of allowing for additional pay without corresponding increases in benefits, which in turn helps stretch limited compensation budgets. Rather than giving across-the-board pay increases (above a cost-of-living adjustment), modest merit increases (an average of 3 percent), or both, which merely add to the base and provide little or no incentive, a true incentive arrangement sets and maintains an adequate and competitive base and provides bonus dollars (that is, a one-time payout per period based strictly on predetermined performance measurements).

Short-Term Incentive Programs

Typically, short-term incentive programs are annual by design, although they can be designed either to include or be limited to shorter durations, with monthly or quarterly objectives. These programs are similar to long-term incentive arrangements in that their objectives are expressed in terms of meaningful and achievable results that can be quantified and verified and that account for organizational and environmental constraints beyond the employee's control.

Historically, annual plans were made available to mid-level and top-level managers to supplement base pay on the basis of individual performance measured against departmental or organizational performance criteria or both. In the past decade or so, short-term incentive programs have become more available to all levels of the work force, as well as more prevalent. It is predicted that the downward extension of short-term programs will be accelerated in the foreseeable future. One important reason for this trend is that short-term incentives by design are driven by the will for organizational survival, especially in today's health care marketplace. Another important reason is that short-term incentives sustain the long-term strategic positioning of the organization via periodic measurement of performance and consequent increments for the achievement of short-term objectives.

It is critical for the success of the short-term incentive program that incentives support specific programs or operating plans or both that in turn are tied to milestones for longer-term objectives. If short-term objectives exist in the absence of long-term objectives or exist with the presence of long-range objectives but are incompatible with such, the organization will surely fail in the attainment of its mission.

If short-term incentives are limited to individual performance, there is potential for a throwback to piecemeal work (that is, "My reward is based totally on what I produce"). By integrating the individual's goals with those of the department and, in turn, the organization, it is more likely that individuals will be motivated to think beyond themselves and appreciate the bigger picture. Integrated short-term incentives foster teamwork and cooperation among employees through formalized communication channels (for example, project teams, quality circles, autonomous work groups, and goal-setting sessions) as well as informal discussions.

In developing a short-term incentive program, the organization must consider a number of factors, such as the determination of critical measures of performance (table 8-2), measurement procedures, realistic target bonuses as percentages of salary, and levels (categories) of work force participation. An example of a typical short-term plan slots designated positions into categories, for example, category I, president/chief executive officer; category II, chief operating officer, chief financial officer; category III, vice presidents; and so forth (table 8-3). Each category is assigned two to five measures of performance critical to its respective areas of responsibility. Incentives are tied to achievement levels predetermined in the setting of realistic objectives associated with performance measurements. Each performance measure includes a *threshold,* the minimal acceptance level of rewardable performance; a *target,* the expected or desired level for reward; and a *maximum,*

Table 8-2. Frequently Used Annual Measures of Performance for Hospitals

Measure	Unit of Measurement
Total discharges	Absolute numbers; indexed
Total admissions	Absolute numbers; indexed
Total expenses	Absolute dollars; percent of budget
Revenue from admission	Absolute dollars; indexed
Cost of admission	Absolute dollars; indexed
Occupancy	Percentage; indexed
Length of stay	Absolute numbers
Total gross revenue	Absolute numbers; percentage of budget
Market share	Percentage
FTEs by occupied bed	Absolute numbers; indexed
Fee class profile	Percentage; indexed
Clinic volume	Absolute numbers; indexed
Accounts receivable	Absolute days
Emergency room visits	Absolute numbers
Net income	Absolute dollars; percentage of total revenue
Gross profit margin	Percentage

Table 8-3. Short-Term Incentive Model (Showing Percentages of Salary)

Category	Below Threshold	Threshold	Target Range	Maximum
I	0	20%	30–40–50%	60%
II	0	15%	22–30–38%	45%
III	0	12%	18–25–32%	38%
IV	0	5%	10–15–20%	25%

the highest reasonable level expected. Payouts are given as a percentage of salary, and because most short-term incentive plans focus on annual results (not day-to-day operations), payment is usually made annually.

Besides the annual plan described, additional or alternative compensation plans should be mentioned in discussing short-term incentives (tables 8-4, 8-5, and 8-6).

- *Lump-Sum Bonuses/Variable Merit:* The typical lump-sum/variable merit payment program is made available to all individuals not covered by any other incentive program in the organization. Distributions are made annually in cash and are made on the basis of organizational performance (for example, net income expressed as a percentage of

Table 8-4. Proportion of Employers Using Alternative Compensation Plans

Strategy	Percent Total	Percent Manufacturers	Percent Services
Profit sharing	32	37	28
Lump-sum bonuses	30	31	29
Individual incentives	28	27	29
Gainsharing	13	20	8
Small-group incentives	14	15	15
All salaried work force	11	13	8
Two-tier pay plan	11	15	7
Pay for knowledge	5	8	2
Earned time off	6	5	7

Source: American Productivity Center/American Compensation Association. *People, Performance, and Pay.* Houston: 1986, p. 29 (abstract).

Table 8-5. Projected Increase in Employers Using Alternative Compensation Plans, 1986–1991

Strategy	Projected Increase
All salaried work force	31%
Pay for knowledge	75%
Gainsharing	68%
Profit sharing	20%
Small-group incentives	70%
Individual incentives	31%
Lump-sum bonuses	29%
Two-tier pay plan	33%
Earned time off	36%

Source: American Productivity Center/American Compensation Association. *People, Performance, and Pay.* Houston: 1986, p. 29 (abstract).

Table 8-6.   Reward and Recognition Alternatives

Method	Motivate Individual	Employer Commitment	Link to Quality and Productivity	Encourage Teamwork
Gainsharing	Medium	High	High	High
Profit sharing	Low	Medium	Low	Medium
Merit pay	High	Medium	High	Low
Lump-sum bonuses	High	Low	High	Low
Recognition programs	Low	Medium	Low	Low
Small-group incentives	Medium	Medium	High	Medium
Individual incentives	High	Medium	High	Low
Noncash rewards	High	Medium	High	Low

Source: American Productivity Center/American Compensation Association. *People, Performance, and Pay.* Houston: 1986, p. 29 (abstract).

total revenue) and not individual performance. The amount each participant receives generally depends on the total amount available for disbursement. The organization may choose to give everyone equal payments regardless of pay level or unequal payments made on a percentage of base pay. Payments should not be discretionary or arbitrary but rather should be consistent and equitable. The bonus payment does not become part of a base wage or salary increase.

- *Profit Sharing:* An annual bonus or a share of the bonus is only paid if the organization's profits increase for the year; the bonus may be received either as cash or on a deferred (retirement) basis. Profit-sharing plans differ from pure productivity sharing plans (such as gainsharing) in that the financial reward is not based on such factors as an individual's sales performance or output per hour but rather on the profit level of the organization as a whole.

- *Gainsharing (Productivity Plan):* In gainsharing plans, rewards are given to a department as a whole and then divided among the employees of that department. Three rather well-known gainsharing plans (Scanlon, Rucker, and Improshare) and several less-known plans (Productivity/Waste Bonus Plans, Group/Plant Plans, and DARCOM) are used in implementing gainsharing programs. Although they differ in some ways, they are similar in that they (1) provide frequent cash bonuses, (2) use production rather than sales-based formulas, and (3) eliminate individual incentive systems. Gainsharing plans include:
  - Scanlon, which has a system of production committees and a screening committee and typically uses a formula that measures the ratio of labor costs to sales dollars
  - Rucker, which uses a suggestion system and productivity committees to enhance performance as measured by value-added productivity formulas; for example, sales value versus the cost of goods sold

- Improshare, which focuses on unit/hour formulas and has no formal involvement structures such as committees but does use and recognize good ideas from employees
- Productivity/Waste Bonus Plans, Group/Plant Plans, and DARCOM, which generally contain no opportunities for employee involvement
- *Small-Group Incentives:* Small-group incentives are similar to gainsharing except bonuses are determined by small-group performance rather than single-formula, unitwide performance. Formulas and bonuses can vary from group to group within a unit, depending on the nature of the work and performance.
- *Pay for Knowledge:* Hourly or salary pay, or pay progression, is determined by the number of jobs an employee can do, not the job(s) he or she actually performs on a given day.
- *Two-Tier Pay Plan:* New hires, as of a certain date, enter at a lower rate of pay than employees previously hired to fill similar jobs prior to that date. This may or may not be part of a collective bargaining agreement. This does not include normal production period practices, automatic pay progression, and so on.
- *Individual Incentives:* All or part of an individual's pay is tied to individual performance. This would include all standard hourly incentive plans, engineered incentives (such as annual or long-term incentives), production incentives, and piece rates. Individual incentives do not include merit raises or executive compensation practices.
- *All Salaried Work Force:* All employees who traditionally would have been considered nonsalaried or hourly in an organizational unit become salaried.
- *Earned Time Off:* For exceptional performance, employees are eligible to earn time off from work with pay.

All short-term incentive plans fall into one of three categories:

- *Discretionary Plan:* Bonus awards are determined by the organization's management (usually on a discretionary and subjective basis).
- *Share of Profit Plan:* Awards are determined by a specific payment formula usually stipulating that a certain amount of profit be paid to participants after some threshold of profits has been reached.
- *Target Incentive Plan:* Incentives are designed to accomplish preset financial and nonfinancial goals and to reward participants to the extent that these goals are achieved.

Noncash Rewards

Everyone enjoys a pat on the back or words of praise for a job well done. After all, people grow up with hugs and kisses as an almost exclusive reinforcer and primary motivator from infancy onward. The imprinting of this non-cash form of reward and recognition remains with us for life as a response mechanism associated with positive achievement. Organizations, like parents, have taken advantage of this sensitivity and capitalized on the opportunities associated with gratifying employees' needs through noncash rewards. Very early on, it becomes apparent that there are always choices, trade-offs, and compromises to be made when satisfying another person's needs.

Organizations have introduced a wide variety of noncash programs designed to recognize employee needs, encourage individual performance and, in turn, organizational performance, and enhance corporate culture. Noncash rewards, for the purposes of this discussion, include benefits, perquisites, and nonfinancial rewards (such as having an office with a view or being assigned to choice committees). Noncash rewards include all the other things an employee receives from the organization besides the dollars on payday. Benefits and perks are, of course, part of the total compensation package, although they are not always viewed as such by employees; benefits and perks are often taken for granted and expected without regard to their cash implications.

Benefits

Benefits usually apply to all employees, whereas perquisites are typically provided to executive management as add-ons to the basic benefits package. During the 1960s, benefits costs rose from approximately 25 percent to 32 percent of direct pay expenditures; today they are roughly 40 percent. Benefits represent a significant amount of money that the organization spends not only in providing for the welfare of its employees, but also in giving something extra as a noncash reward for employees' efforts to foster organizational growth. With such large expenditures associated with benefits costs, the organization must consider which benefits are to be offered, who is eligible, who participates, when benefits are received, and what the level of copayments, if any, will be. Most organizations offer a core or basic benefits package; other benefits may be added to enrich the package. Examples of core, or basic, benefits include:

- Medical/dental insurance
- Short-term disability
- Holidays/sick days/paid time off
- Vacation time
- Basic group life insurance
- Pension plan
- Profit sharing, 401(k) plans, tax-sheltered annuity (TSA)

Examples of add-on benefits include:

- Vision care
- Pharmacy discounts

- Annual physical examinations
- Long-term disability
- Supplemental life insurance
- Travel/accident insurance
- Leaves of absence
- Parking
- Educational reimbursement
- Unemployment compensation
- U.S. savings bonds
- Funeral pay
- Blood bank
- Time off or pay for jury days
- Employee assistance program
- Cafeteria discounts
- Uniforms
- Lockers
- Discount tickets
- Credit union
- Group auto insurance
- Child care
- Professional dues
- Flexible spending account (Section 125, IRS), in which an employee can place a limited amount of pretax earnings to be spent later for certain benefits (such as vision care or child care)

Perquisites

The Deficit Reduction Act of 1984 (DEFRA) and the Tax Reform Act of 1986 significantly affected the attractiveness of offering certain nontaxable benefits. Careful consideration, interpretation, and understanding of the Internal Revenue Service Code should be taken into account in determining the inclusion or exclusion of the following examples as taxable or nontaxable (perquisite) benefits.

- Company car; chauffeur
- Parking
- Air travel (first class, company plane, special business travel accident insurance)
- Club membership (dinner clubs, athletic or health clubs, and so forth)
- Financial counseling
- Legal counseling
- Supplemental medical coverage (periodic or annual physical examinations)
- Supplemental group life insurance
- Supplemental retirement plans

- Personal computer
- Sports and theater tickets
- Home entertainment
- Dining facilities
- Sabbaticals
- Discounted products
- Executive training programs
- Dependent tuition reimbursement
- Physical fitness programs
- Outplacement
- Credit cards, company accommodations for vacation use, yacht, security devices, bodyguard, liability insurance, employment contract, post-retirement consulting agreement

Nonfinancial Rewards

Nonfinancial rewards is a catchall term for those things companies offer as a way to reward or recognize employees nonfinancially. Some rewards are more tangible than others. Examples of nonfinancial rewards include the following:

- *MBO (management by objectives) prototype:* Employees are involved in negotiating standards against which performance is measured.
- *Earned time off:* Employees are allowed more leisure time; once production standards are met, they may leave work (pay is based on production, not hours).
- *Flextime:* Employees' needs for varying time schedules are recognized (there is usually a core time when all employees must be present).
- *Labor/management committees:* Union and management come together to solve commonly agreed-upon problems.
- *Quality of work life programs (QWL):* QWL programs are focus groups or quality circles (patterned after the Japanese *sho-shudan-kauri* system where employees voluntarily work with managers in small groups to improve productivity and quality).

Examples of tangible nonfinancial rewards include:

- Service awards (pens, watches, and so forth)
- Employee appreciation day
- An office with one or more of the following: walls, a door, a window, matching furniture, size larger than 10 × 10 feet, carpet, closet, or bookshelves
- A secretary
- Personalized stationery
- Change to a more meaningful title
- Keys to the lavatory

Long-Term Incentive Programs

Long-term incentive programs usually have two- to five-year time horizons related to objectives, with payouts staggered over that time period. Unlike short-term incentive programs, which are typically measured on an annual basis, paid in cash (though deferred payment may be an option), and offered to participants below senior management, long-term incentives are usually paid on a deferred compensation basis, and participation is restricted to top-level management. The objectives for the programs are often set by the board of directors in concert with the executives (or vice versa) and reflect the specific interests of that top level in the development of the organizational mission. Because the programs are long term by design, the objectives reflect a gradual means (compared with short-term objectives) to reach these longer-term organizational objectives. An assumption in developing long-term incentive programs is that the higher up in the organization one goes, the more responsibility one assumes; and with greater responsibility comes greater risk at a higher visibility. By limiting the number of persons participating in the plan, top-level management can focus more sharply on the direction taken by the organization and thus minimize risks.

Three general types of deferred compensation are associated with long-term incentive programs.

- *Stock Option:* The executive is given an option to buy stock at a fixed price within a defined period of time. The stocks are taxed at favorable capital gains rates if certain qualifications are met. The executive must invest his or her own money, and the stock appreciates with the success of the organization.
- *Stock Award:* The executive is given the right to a variable number of shares, depending on defined performance criteria. The value of the stock is taxed as ordinary income.
- *Performance Units/Phantom Shares:* The executive is given the right to several performance units that vary with the defined performance criteria. This plan is similar to stock awards, although it is not affected by stock market fluctuations. The value of the units appreciates with the success of the organization.

As with any plan design, some critical issues and questions must be addressed. This is particularly evident with long-term incentive plans because of the legal and tax implications associated with capital accumulation (figure 8-5). For example, stock options have been the most popular long-term incentive because they can be taxed as capital gains, but that advantage no longer exists since the 1986 tax code revisions.

Conclusion

Whether inherent to the personality or learned through experience, reward and recognition are primary motivators for goal attainment. We are naturally

Figure 8-5.   Long-Term Incentive Compensation Considerations

- Is executive stock ownership important?
- Should the executive be required to make a personal investment in the stock?
- Should the plan relate to the stock's fair market value or to the ownership of the stock?
- Should the payout relate to the company's financial results instead of stock market performances
- What is the impact on the company's financial statements? Earnings per share?
- Should the plan be approved by shareholders?
- Does the corporate law of the state in which the company is incorporated permit the plan design?
- Is the stock publicly traded and registered? If not, how is the stock to be valued?
- Does the Securities and Exchange Commission require the plan to be registered?
- What special rules apply to insiders?
- What are the tax effects to the participants? To the company?
- What are the accounting implications?
- What must be disclosed to shareholders?

enticed and oftentimes driven by the carrot dangling at the end of the stick. The perceived value and rate at which we go after that carrot is determined by the nature and extent to which a need must be satisfied.

The organization's prosperity hinges on its ability to manipulate recognition and reward to maximize employee satisfaction and organizational demands. Today, organizations are moving more toward pay-for-performance programs, recognizing that not only is money the key motivation but that people are motivated to do more and do it better if they see a direct relationship between their effort and its outcomes. In addition, organizations increasingly are coming to appreciate that noncash rewards can be equally meaningful to employees and can be primary motivators.

References

American Productivity Center. *Reward Systems and Productivity: A Fiscal Report for the White House Conference on Productivity.* Houston: American Productivity Centers, 1983, pp. 1–16.

Burda, D. IRS ruling clears way for incentive pay plans. *Modern Healthcare* 18(7):38–39, Feb. 12, 1988.

Crystal, G. S., and Silbermann, S. J. Outlook on compensation and benefits. *Personnel* 63(4):7–10, Apr. 1986.

Dudley, G. W., and Goodson, S. I. *Psychology of Call Reluctance.* Dallas: Behavioral Science Research Press, 1986, pp. 1–192.

Fitzgerald, K. The right rewards guarantee better workers. *Savings Institutions,* Feb. 1988, pp. 43–60.

Gardner, E. Benefits managers undermined by need to contain costs. *Modern Healthcare* 17:41–50, Mar. 27, 1987.

Incentive program sharpens executives' performance. *Hospitals* 57(17):37–38, Sept. 1983.

King, P. *Performance Planning and Appraisal.* Chicago: McGraw-Hill, 1984, p. 160.

Lutz, S. Hospitals upgrading benefits to gain competitor advantage. *Modern Healthcare* 17:54, Mar. 27, 1987.

Paine, T. H. What's in store for compensation and benefits: 1986 and beyond. *Compensation and Benefits Manager,* Winter 1986, pp. 85–90.

Platt, H. D., and McCarthy, D. J. Executive compensation: performance and patience. *Business Horizons,* Jan.–Feb. 1985, pp. 48–53.

Rowland, D. C., and Greene, B. Incentive pay: productivity's own reward. *Personnel Journal* 66(3):48–57, Mar. 1987.

Shyavitz, L., Rosenbloom, D., and Conover, L. Financial incentives for middle managers. *HCM (Health Care Management) Review* 10(3):37–44, Summer 1985.

Spencer Research Reports. Incentive compensation growing in health care field. Chicago: Charles D. Spencer and Associates, Apr. 10, 1987, p. 6.

Umbdenstock, R. J., and Hageman, W. M. *Hospital Corporate Leadership: The Board and Chief Executive Officer Relationship.* Chicago: American Hospital Publishing, Inc., 1984.

Weil, P. A., and Wesbury, S. A. CEO evaluation in the 1980s. *Trustee* 37(8):27–29, Aug. 1984.

Wenke, P. C. 13 steps toward enhancing productivity. *Hospitals* 57(19):109–12, Oct. 1, 1983.

Whitted, G. S., and Ewell, C. M. A survey of hospital management incentive programs. *Hospitals* 58(5):90–94, Mar. 1, 1984.

The Wyatt Company. Defined benefit plans that look like defined contribution plans. *Personnel Journal* 65(2):103–9, Feb. 1986.

Annotated Bibliography

Arvey, R. D. *Fairness in Selecting Employees.* Reading, MA: Addison-Wesley Publishing Co., 1979.

This basic primer summarizes pertinent litigation for the layperson.

Berger, R., and Hart, T. *Statistical Process Control — A Guide for Implementation.* New York City: Marcel Dekker, Inc. (ASQC Quality Press), 1986.

This guide provides introductory material on the application of statistical process control techniques. Statistical concepts and techniques with examples are presented, as are guidelines on how to conduct process capability studies. The use of "X" and R charts (sample averages and ranges) are reviewed with specific case examples.

Block, P. *The Empowered Manager: Positive Political Skills at Work.* San Francisco: Jossey-Bass, 1987.

Block's book is a very easy to read book that discusses the implications of culture on performance. The author details two major options that are available. The first is a bureaucratic organization, which has certain limits on individual performance. The second is an empowered organization that has as part of its mission working with employees and getting them enrolled in the vision of greatness. Block provides useful exercises for the reader. His section on creating and communicating a vision of greatness is excellent.

Burda, D. IRS ruling clears way for incentive pay plans. *Modern Healthcare* 18(7):38–39, Feb. 12, 1988.

According to the most recent IRS ruling, IRS attorneys said that a reasonable incentive compensation program determined by hospital net income doesn't jeopardize a not-for-profit hospital's tax status. This IRS ruling lifts the last major obstacle preventing not-for-profit hospitals from initiating incentive compensation for all employees. To have a plan approved by the IRS, a hospital should document that an incentive pay plan has a valid business purpose linked to the hospital mission, that is, designed to improve the quality of patient care, reduce unnecessary costs, or recruit valuable employees.

Cascio, W. F. *Costing Human Resources: The Financial Impact of Behavior in Organizations.* New York City: Van Nostrand Reinhold Co., 1982.

The "return on investment" discussion is interesting and familiar to human resources professionals who follow J. Fitz-enz and agree with his efforts regarding return on investment standards for human resources departments.

Eastaugh, S. R. Improving hospital productivity under PPS: managing cost reductions. *Hospital and Health Services Administration* 30(4):97–111, July–Aug. 1985.

This timely article presents a three-stage approach to productivity improvement within a health care institution. Stage I is defined as an assessment stage, where tasks are defined and staffing ratios are developed. Stage II uses the information from stage I to schedule patients as well as resources. Stage III deals with the issue of incentives. The author systematically ties these concepts to institutional productivity management.

Garrett, L. J., and Silver, M. *Production Management Analysis.* New York City: Harcourt, Brace and World, Inc., 1966.

This is a detailed presentation of industrial engineering techniques, including queuing theory, inventory control, and time and motion analysis.

Goldberg, A. J. *Hospital Departmental Profiles.* Chicago: American Hospital Publishing, Inc., 1986.

This is a thorough review of the operational parameters of the major hospital departments.

Hansen, B. *Quality Control: Theory and Applications.* Englewood Cliffs, NJ: Prentice-Hall, 1963.

As stated in the preface, this book was designed for use in introductory and intermediate courses in engineering and management. It was also written for use as a working reference for quality assurance managers, engineers, technicians, and other persons working in quality control and related fields. The objective of the book was as follows: to set forth the fundamentals of statistical and economic analysis, to provide many applications, and to give adequate source material for further study. The primary shortcoming of this book is that most of the material is geared toward the manufacturing industry.

Holly, W. H., and Hubert, S. F. Will your performance appraisal system hold up in court? *Personnel* 59(1):59–64, Jan.–Feb. 1982.

Human resources managers can measure the vulnerability of their performance appraisal systems by comparing them with ones involved in discrimination suits. This article summarizes the findings and analyses of 66 court cases involving alleged discrimination caused by the use (or misuse) of performance appraisals. On the basis of these findings, the authors provide recommendations that may help employers successfully defend themselves if a discrimination charge or suit is brought against them.

Johannides, D. F. *Cost Containment through Systems Engineering.* Germantown, MD: Aspen Systems Corp., 1979.

The author discusses how to integrate systems engineering into the hospital management strategy.

Mintzberg, H. *Structures in Fives: Designing Effective Organizations.* Englewood Cliffs, NJ: Prentice-Hall, Inc., 1983.

Mintzberg does not offer employee selection and assessment tools, but his organizational design theory is worthy of study and consideration. In particular, readers should contemplate the organization design concept he calls the "machine bureaucracy" and its fatal flaws when applied in knowledge industries.

Odiorne, G. S. *Strategic Management of Human Resources.* San Francisco: Jossey-Bass, 1984.

Odiorne explores human resources as assets and provides some discussion of "portfolio analysis" techniques.

Rosander, A. C. *Applications of Quality Control in the Service Industries.* New York City and Basel: Marcel Dekker, Inc. (ASQC Quality Press), 1985.

As this author points out, although quality control started in the factory, its application is just as important in the service industries. He further states that applying quality control most effectively to service industries requires an analysis of the unique characteristics of service operations, the role of the buyer as well as that of the seller, and the application of appropriate quality concepts and techniques. In Part I, "Service Industry Applications," the Health Services chapter provides, via actual case material, some very good application material for the average manager. The remaining two parts of the book, "Statistics" and "Techniques," build upon the case material and provide enough technical material for someone to develop and install their first quality control system.

Rowland, D. C., and Greene, B. Incentive pay: productivity's own reward. *Personnel Journal* 66(3):48–57, Mar. 1987.

According to the authors, incentive plans can make an important contribution to profitability and the retention of key personnel because they tie compensation directly to productivity. To achieve these benefits, however, the plan must be well designed. Bonus programs, group incentives, and commission plans are discussed as well as six basic issues for consideration in the development of a plan: what business goals need to be accomplished, who should participate, how results should be measured, how much should be paid, what level of performance is expected, and how rewards should be distributed.

Sahney, V. K. Managing variability in demand: a strategy for productivity improvement in health care services. *HCM (Health Care Management) Review* 7(2):37–41, Spring 1982.

Health care institutions often face demands for services that fluctuate monthly, daily, or even by the hour. Health care services cannot be produced and stored for later delivery. This article presents a variety of strategies that can be used effectively to manage the variability in demand that health care institutions experience.

Sashkin, M. Appraising appraisal: ten lessons from research for practice. *Organizational Dynamics*, Winter 1981, pp. 37–50.

Legal and pragmatic considerations require that organizations analyze their overall performance appraisal systems, not simply their performance appraisal techniques. The author encourages the reader to examine the overall picture of performance appraisal and characterize the system as a whole. Ten "rule of thumb" guidelines are presented, including asking such questions as, "Are job descriptions as specific job goal documents based on behavioral or job-relevant performance standards?" and "Do appraisal sessions have a problem-solving focus?" These guidelines should help readers to focus on correcting existing appraisal system problems, redesigning the system, or changing one's own personal appraisal behaviors or procedures.

Schein, E. *Organizational Culture and Leadership.* San Francisco: Jossey-Bass, 1985.

If you were to read just one book regarding the topic of corporate culture, Schein's book would be the one to read. There are significant discussions on the foundation of culture, what culture is all about, and the relationship of culture to leadership. One important concept in the book is that the key role of a leader is to manage the corporate culture of his or her organization.

Schermerhorn, J. R. Improving health care productivity through high performance managerial development. *HCM (Health Care Management) Review* 12(4):49–56, Fall 1987.

This article presents a systematic approach to developing a high-performance team. Three key elements of productivity—ability, support, and effort—are discussed in the context of developing this team.

Schneier, C. E., Beatty, R. W., and Baird, L. S. How to construct a successful performance appraisal system. *Training and Development Journal* 40(4):38–42, Apr. 1986.

The authors state that persons designing, implementing, evaluating, and using performance appraisal systems in organizations must realize that such systems cannot be successful unless they are consistent with the realities of the managerial work and organizational environments. Appraisal systems fail for a variety of reasons, centering on such problem areas as measurement (deciding what to evaluate), judgment (deciding how to appraise), policy (using the results of the appraisal), and organization (recognizing how managers work and assessing the organization's culture). An increasing number of organizations have found that appraisal systems are effective if they enhance the superior-subordinate relationship by allowing for frequent communication, specifications of expectations, accurate evaluations, and problem solving.

Shyavitz, L., Rosenbloom, D., and Conover, L. Financial incentives for middle managers. *HCM (Health Care Management) Review* 10(3):37–44, Summer 1985.

This article describes and evaluates an attempt to build a management incentive system in a large public hospital. The results show that, even in as complicated an environment as a public, inner-city, highly unionized teaching hospital, it is possible to establish and run an incentive program with financial rewards for performance. Narrative discussions as well as schematics are presented to highlight the objectives and features of the management incentive program. On the basis of their findings, the authors suggest that incentive programs more traditionally associated with the investor-owned sector can work in not-for-profit settings, if structured properly.

Smalley, H. E., and Freeman, J. R. *Hospital Industrial Engineering.* New York City: Harcourt, Brace and World, Inc., 1966.

The authors offer a general discussion of systems engineering techniques applicable to the health care industry.

Taylor, M. S., and Sackheim, K. K. Graphology. *Personnel Administrator* 33(5):71–76, May 1988.

Although the expected skepticism of the academic is present, this presentation of graphology suggests that it might be applicable to the health care setting, if used properly and not utilized as the sole predictor of employee suitability.

Tomasko, R. M. *Downsizing: Reshaping the Corporation for the Future.* New York City: AMACOM (a division of the American Management Association), 1987.

The author discusses how to flatten the organization's structure and distinguishes between "control staff" and "support staff."

Walker, J. W. *Human Resources Planning.* New York City: McGraw-Hill Book Co., 1980.

Pragmatic and well-organized, Walker's book makes it clear that human resources planning is a management process, not merely a personnel function. He defines the work of the management process.